The Book of Judo

also published as *The Art of Peace*

George Ohsawa

George Ohsawa Macrobiotic Foundation
Chico, California

Other books by George Ohsawa in English include: *Acupuncture and the Philosophy of the Far East; Atomic Age and the Philosophy of the Far East; Cancer and the Philosophy of the Far East; Essential Ohsawa; Gandhi, the Eternal Youth; Jack and Mitie; Macrobiotic Guidebook for Living; Macrobiotics: An Invitation to Health and Happiness; Order of the Universe; Philosophy of Oriental Medicine; Practical Guide to Far Eastern Macrobiotic Medicine; Unique Principle; You Are All Sanpaku;* and *Zen Macrobiotics.* Contact the publisher at the address below for a complete list of available titles.

This book is made possible through a generous donation from Holistic Holiday at Sea.

Translated by William Gleason
Edited by Sandy Rothman
Keyboarded by Alice Salinero
Text layout and design by Carl Ferré
Cover design by Carl Campbell

Published as *Le Livre du Judo* in French (Paris)	1952
English Edition	1990
Current Printing: edited and reformatted	2011 Jan 29

© copyright 1990 by
George Ohsawa Macrobiotic Foundation
  PO Box 3998, Chico, California 95927-3998
  530-566-9765; fax 530-566-9768
  www.ohsawamacrobiotics.com; gomf@ohsawamacrobiotics.com

Published with the help of East West Center for Macrobiotics
  www.eastwestmacrobiotics.com

Library of Congress Catalog Card Number: 90-32077
ISBN 978-0-918860-50-7

Publisher's Note

I am very happy this book has finally been translated into English and published, about 40 years after George Ohsawa lectured on this subject just after World War II.

The Book of Judo has also been titled *The Art of Peace* because the real aim of all the martial ways, including judo and aikido, is maintaining peace. What Ohsawa basically discusses in this book is not the techniques of judo or aikido, although he began by writing on the founders of both arts. What Ohsawa wants to discuss here is the cause or causes of war and how to realize peace on earth. Why did he want to relate judo and aikido with the establishment of world peace? In order to explain this, I have to tell you a little about the background of this book.

Around 1950, five years after the end of the World War II, I was going to Ohsawa's school, Maison Ignoramus, in Tokyo to study macrobiotics. One morning Ohsawa gave a lecture based on his new book, *Le Livre du Judo*. Having lost the war, Japan had lost everything—industries and businesses as well as its way of life and beliefs: the meaning of life, home, and nation which the Japanese people were so proud of. As a result, confusion prevailed. People didn't know what to do except obtain food through the black market or earn money by selling military goods on the black market.

In those confused times, Ohsawa taught macrobiotics at his center. One day he met the renowned aikido master Morihei Ueshiba at his *dojo* because, by coincidence, Ueshiba's *dojo* was located very close to Ohsawa's school. Ohsawa highly admired Master Ueshiba and recommended that everybody learn aikido because the principle of aikido is not fighting but rather turning the enemy into a friend. This was also Ohsawa's principle. For this reason, many Japanese macrobiotic followers became aikido disciples, especially among those who went to live in Europe. One of these was Seigo Yamaguchi, head instructor at the Aikido Dojo in Shinjuku, Tokyo. He was the first of Ohsawa's students living at the center to begin studying aikido. William Gleason, who first translated this book into English, is an American disciple of Seigo Yamaguchi.

Ohsawa understood the spirit of aikido from Master Ueshiba— the concept of changing an enemy into a friend. This understanding and his meeting Ueshiba must be what inspired Ohsawa to write this book.

Ohsawa also wanted to explain the Far Eastern "primitive mentality" at a time when Japan was rebuilding its culture and economy, and he did so in this book. World Federalism was, of course, aiming to establish world peace, and Ohsawa's version was based on macrobiotic spiritual and dietary principles. In reality, he united himself with the movement so that he could easily distribute macrobiotic ideas to the people of Japan who, more than any one, wanted peace in the world. *The Book of Judo* was written under such circumstances.

"Judo is, above all, a cooperative activity where those who are opposed to each other are united by the common goal of polishing themselves as well as bringing each other to perfection through actual training," wrote Ohsawa. "Neither peace nor freedom can be established by the elimination of the other side."

Since that time, nearly 40 years have passed. The world has experienced great peace, but it was not real peace. It was a peace protected by atomic bombs and nuclear weapons. It was a peace controlled by a winner's tyranny. Such exclusive one-person governments started to fall last year in Europe when many countries turned towards democratic governments. This is the first step to world peace. Ohsawa's *The Book of Judo* is a guiding light showing the causes of war and the way to establish true peace, spiritually and physically, starting from the individual. At a time when the world is showing signs of establishing the unification of opposites, in other words, turning towards peace, I highly recommend reading this book. I think this is one of Ohsawa's greatest books. He prepared well for the topics he selected.

We chose Mr. Gleason as the translator because he stayed in Japan for several years studying aikido and macrobiotics and is now a fifth degree black belt teaching in Boston. He translated from the Japanese text with the help of his wife Hisako, a Japanese macrobiotic student. I appreciate their work every much. I would also like to thank Sandy Rothman for his thorough editing, Carl Ferré for text design and production, and Carl Campbell for designing the beautiful cover.

Herman Aihara, President
George Ohsawa
Macrobiotic Foundation
April 1990

Contents

Preface

Judo is an art. It is different from activities that fall under the category of sports. It is a practical, aesthetic, physical, and psychological art. More than a means of self-defense, it should fall under the category of an art of adaptability, one of the functions of instinct.

The adaptability of human beings is truly amazing. Our ability to adapt grows and develops in a thousand different ways. Real medicine, government, economy, education, and theory are similar to judo or aikido. They are all special characteristics of our instinctive adaptability.

If adaptability is a special characteristic of instinct, then in order to develop it the most important thing is to understand what instinct is. There is no branch of science capable of explaining either the laws that govern instinct or the mechanism of instinct. Therefore, there is no education, economics, government, or medicine that is true—that is to say, unique and eternal. All these institutions are relative, limited, and temporary teachings that are constantly in a state of flux. Little by little they are all going towards their own dissolution. If a particular religion or way of medicine outlasts the others, this is proof that it has a more deeply rooted perception of human instinct. Modern Christianity is a fossilized example of this and Buddhism is another. Oriental medicine, although relatively unknown in the West, is flourishing and respected by some 400 million Chinese as well as the Japanese (who are the most Westernized people in the Far East). Some eighty years ago in Japan, Oriental medicine was completely suppressed and stamped out. Compared to the original, that which has been revived today is little more than amateurism. The doctors of herbal medicine today are totally ignorant of Oriental medicine. In spite of this, the degree of respect that Oriental medicine receives is really amazing. Real Oriental medicine is already obscure. Those who practice it today depend on pieces of information they can pick up from old books.

From the time Western civilization was imported, the once peaceful Japan, represented by the paintings of Hiroshige and Utamaro,[1] has been turned upside down. The true judo could no longer survive. One is reminded of the story of the pitiful crow who threw away his feathers, thinking he could borrow those of the peacock. It was believed that the rifle could replace judo and kendo. It is obvious that, even at that time, judo was already thought of as no more than an art of self-defense.

Judo, however, is not so simplistic. It is both spiritual and physical, hence philosophical and physiological. It is a method of gaining intuitive understanding of the mechanism of adaptability. If this understanding is given practical application, our instinct as well as our willpower are strengthened. It is not like that conceptual or scientific knowledge that obscures instinct. As with all the ancient teachings of the Far East, judo is straightforward, direct, and doesn't depend on any use of special or complex tools or instruments. There are no detailed explanations. Rather, the focus is on how to establish and strengthen instinct, which is the source of our power of understanding, judgment, and will. At the *dojo* (the practice hall where the *do* is studied), students practice together under the critical eye of the master who is preparing them for future physical, spiritual, and also biological battles. There are many *dojos* everywhere, and there are many teachers here and there who make their living by teaching judo or kendo. Unfortunately, those who deserve the title of *shihan*, or master, are very rare.

Jigoro Kano, credited as the founder of judo, was such a master. He did not sell his techniques or his ability. He reformed and unified various styles of jujitsu, which had degenerated. The morality of judo depreciates constantly because some who want to learn it are unhappy people who believe in the use of force and hope to conquer the tangible world of data. Secondly, it takes a long time and a lot of practice, with little explanation, in order to really grasp the unwavering and unifying principle that is the barometer of humanity and the only path towards the kingdom of heaven.

Accordingly, judo was called the school that teaches nothing. Kano succeeded in creating a new school of judo called Kodokan. After his death, there was no one to replace him. The tendency here towards degeneration is all too obvious. Being too busy with reformation, reconstruction, and propaganda, he had no time to deepen and spread his own understanding of the principle of judo. Some twenty years prior, Kano *sensei* (teacher) had sent his best student, Minoru Mochizuki, to study aikido with Master Morihei Ueshiba. Here we should pause and take note of a very important point. A great master like Kano at seventy years of age wanted to begin studying another art, which he found superior to his own. This flexible mentality itself is the main characteristic of the principle of judo. It is also the traditional character of the samurai period of Japan that made possible the unification of the various schools of jujitsu. Ueshiba is already a free man of seventy. He continues to pass his time doing exactly as he chooses. Furthermore, he requires no special instrument to accomplish his dreams. A free person has no fear. One needs no weapons and does not immobilize an opponent with physical strength, but with that love that automatically changes the enemy into a good friend. Ueshiba sensei was the last and probably the greatest master in the history of Japanese *budo*.

Mochizuki studied aikido under Ueshiba for several years and earned the grade of eighth *dan* (degree) black belt. He became one of Ueshiba's top students. He is, at the same time, also a sixth *dan* in Kodokan judo. On February 2, 1951 he left for Paris on the steamer La Marseillaise, with three of his students, as an official representative of aikido. He was sponsored by the Society for the New Japanese Culture (*Shin Nihon Bunka Kyokai*) and the Japanese branch of the Association of World Federalists (*Sekai Renpo Kyokai Nihon Shibu*). He wanted to show that aikido is a physical, physiological, and spiritual application of the unique principle of Far Eastern philosophy and science and that, as such, it is also the foundation of the world's three great religions. He wanted to show that it is a road to peace. Mochizuki was unable to put all of this into words, but he illustrated it by his own being and countenance.

Since neither Mochizuki nor his master explained the scientific aspects of the true meaning of judo, I will attempt to do so in their place. My ability in Western language is extremely limited and so I cannot explain the physiological, philosophical, and other scientific aspects in great detail. Nevertheless, I am overjoyed to have, at last, this opportunity to explain primitive mentality, as I promised Professor Lévy-Bruhl twenty years ago. I am sure it is worthwhile to do so for the establishment of a deeper understanding between East and West.

According to Lao Tsu, those who are free can accomplish all their dreams, at any time and to whatever degree they choose, without the need for any external tool or implement. Freedom, then, is the name given to the actions of those who do whatever they desire and as much as they desire, forever. Happiness is the internal state of such people. Judo is one of the special activities of those who have attained freedom and happiness.

Introduction

This book, written by one primitive man, is an exposition of the term "primitive mentality" as used in the title of several books written by Dr. Lucien Lévy-Bruhl, the late president of the French Philosophical Society.[2] In spite of his study, the real meaning of this term was a total enigma to him. After reading his book, I promised the professor that I would write a commentary to elucidate the real meaning of this term. After twenty years of preparation, I have, at last, been able to fulfill my promise to him by writing *The Book of Judo* [retitled *The Art of Peace* in the first English edition]. At the same time, this book is also an attempt to show the underlying foundations of a civilization that made it possible for Japan to live for many years in peace and freedom. It is, furthermore, an attempt to simply and clearly point out to the Western world the pitiable fate of a people uprooted from their own native civilization.

A people uprooted from their maternal civilization, like a stem without any roots, must sooner or later perish. This is the very reason for the unprecedented defeat of Japan in World War II.

Japan was too quick to throw away its own culture and adopt that of outside countries. The Japanese seemed to view those other civilizations as more beautiful and powerful. However, this was not the case at all. It was merely a fascination with the contrast presented by a completely different kind of civilization, a civilization exactly the opposite of their own, that brought this about.

The defeat or decline of an indigenous nation results mainly from its people forgetting or denying their own roots and foundations. Yet it is only natural that people confined to one place for too long a period of time will, sooner or later, develop a feeling of monotony and desire a change in their way of life. This is a physical, physiological, and sociological law. This very same law explains the affinity of the chemical elements to each other as well as the decomposition of chemical compounds into their various basic elements. It is a common characteristic of all things to seek their exact opposite—for example, that which seems exotic, original, or ideal in the opposite sex.

In the case where a certain individual seems to be more attractive than others, it is necessarily because he or she appears youthful, happier, healthier, and more like a child who knows no fear. It can also be said that this person is probably less shrewd or clever than others. On the other hand, those who are more conservative will be more flexible in their thinking and will seem older.

People who dislike those whose natures are opposite or different from their own are incapable of any quality of emotion beyond that of self-love. They are solitary, isolated egoists without friends. Their hatred, contempt, and fear are signs of their unhappiness. Such people are, in reality, already dead. They are already, even at this present moment, living in hell. They lack all the various elements of happiness. Those who are without friends do not know how to live. Those who have enemies cannot become as the child who knows no fear. As stated in the Old Testament, "If one falls, the other can lift his companion up again; but woe betide the solitary person who when down has no partner to help him up" (Ecclesiastes 4:10).[3] They are defeated before the battle begins. They have no alternative but to live as slaves to the invisible master known as fear. The only freedom they possess is created in their own minds. It is imaginary and illusory.

In any case, it has been twenty years since my first publications in French—*The Unique Principle; The Book of Flowers;* and *Acupuncture in Chinese Medicine.* Now, I am extremely happy to present this book. The same thread of truth and meaning runs through all of my books. Namely, to present in an altogether new form the origins and sources of an ancient civilization that no longer exists.

This is to help establish a new and unified culture for all of humanity.

There would be no greater joy for me than to hear your most frank and candid criticisms of this book. I must say, however, that if you truly desire to discover great polarity such as that existing between man and woman, or if you wish to discover not only the practical utility but even the precious value of the smallest thing, such as a basic particle of matter in this world of relativity, you must first of all be a person of sound mind and healthy body. Lacking psychological and physiological health, you will find nothing.

Above and beyond your respect and admiration for judo, the weaponless art developed from jujitsu, above all you must be healthy. The health of which I speak, and which is also indicated by the medicine of the Far East, is something quite different from what you may imagine. I have never been able to respect or confide in someone who does not have good health. I do not take seriously the opinions or judgments of an unhealthy person. Even if you declare that you are healthy, I cannot easily believe you because my standard of measure is a unique one. If you are not in good health, then I hope you will attempt to really grasp the underlying principles of judo of which I am going to speak in this book.

Tao, do, or *michi* are Japanese terms for way, or method, and are part of words such as the art of *judo,* the flexible way; *kendo,* the way of the sword; *ido,* the way of medicine; *shodo,* the way of calligraphy; *kado,* the way of poetry, and other traditional arts. These appear to be different, but, in reality, they are all only different approaches to grasping the one principle that leads to the unified world of peace and freedom. When this principle of principles is grasped, we gain the ability to realize our dreams without the use of any tool, instrument, or weapon. This is the ability that defines true health and, at the same time, is the world of the true human being, the sage.

If you are able to fulfill the following six conditions, you are fully qualified to criticize this book:

1. No fatigue.
2. Good appetite.

3. Good sleep.

4. Excellent memory.

5. Good humor.

6. *Sunao:* A gentle nature combined with inner strength. (*Sunao* is the ability to make balance and harmony with both the physical and the spiritual worlds. This covers the three fundamental strengths: physiological, psychological, and spiritual.)

This is a self-consultation. The first three conditions are physiological (10 points each); the last three are psychological (4th and 5th are 20 points each, 6th is 30 points). If you score more than 40 points, you are passably healthy; 60 points, you are in good health; 80 points, excellent health.

However, let's check the meaning of each category more closely.

1. No fatigue means a state of health in which one does not catch even one cold a year. Nearsightedness; astigmatism; color blindness; irregular, difficult, or prolonged menstruation (more than three days); baldness or prematurely white hair are not the problems of a healthy person. If you lack the vitality of a lion suddenly attacking a rabbit in your work (reading, walking, calculating, or solving difficult problems), this is a sign of profound fatigue.

2. A good appetite means that you can always relish any simple dish. A simple bowl of soup with a few vegetables or a little bread and cheese bring you great pleasure and satisfaction.

3. Good sleep means that you are able to fall asleep anytime or anyplace within three minutes of laying your head down, not stirring during your sleep, and awakening exactly at the time you have fixed. You sleep so deeply that you have no need for more than six hours of sleep. In no case do you ever sleepwalk or dream, especially speaking or weeping dreams. The only exception is a true and prophetic dream. This is a sign of good health.

4. Good memory. Even if you appear to be strong and robust, if you lack a sharp memory, you are already in a dangerous state. The

brain cells are already dead or degenerating.

5. A person of good humor is one whose presence is like a flower on the open plains. Your presence alone makes others feel joyful, and they begin to say things that make each other feel good.

6. Someone with *sunao* is of a gentle but firm nature and appears smart, chic, elegant, and noble. You are kind and calm. Reserved in appearance, inside you are firm, just, and free.

How many points have you scored for your health?

Generally speaking, one should be able to get a good grade on these six points without any special method or training, just as all plants and animals in nature are able to do. These six conditions can be established through macrobiotics,[4] by adjusting one's daily food and drink. This is a natural way of healing that can relieve both physiological and psychological illnesses. It is the physiological, philosophical application of nature's principle.

The foundation of judo is the macrobiotic way of diet, a diet like that of Jesus. Macrobiotics provides the key to solving all food problems which are, in fact, the very root of international conflicts. This holds true whether they are problems of territorial dispute or whether they occur within commercial food companies. Because macrobiotics preserves a brilliant state of health without the need for expensive and heavy animal protein, it may help solve many socio-medical, economic, political, and philosophical problems.

The principle of judo is one kind of philosophy. It is, in fact, a matrix of science and philosophy. It is a basis for mutual understanding and, therefore, provides us with a basis for a world government constitution. Furthermore, as it is also the basis of the world's three great religions, it gives us a standpoint from which to judge human behavior, ideology, and technology.

Judo is not a sport. It is neither an art of attack nor an art of defense. It is not a way of knocking someone down with superior force such as wrestling or boxing. It is not a means of attack and defense with weapons. Judo does not compete for superiority of weight, muscle, or technique such as is the case with skiing, swimming, or diving. Fish and birds are far superior to human beings in these abilities. Judo is a method through which each individual can use his or her freedom to develop a happy life. Judo teaches us how to live in this world.

That is to say:

- Judo teaches us respect for everyone, especially those who attack us with force or other means. They point out our mistakes and weak points and help us to study and progress.
- Judo also shows us the superiority of calm and gentility, which overrides the profound strength of constitutions and personalities.
- Through quick and practical movements that require judgment, reasoning, and instant action, judo nurtures willpower, instinct, intuition, and adaptability.
- Finally, judo forces us to intuitively grasp the dialectic conception of this world and the order of the universe, which are the basis of a strategy of peace for establishing a society of free people.

Furthermore, judo is a method that teaches how people can live in eternal happiness without fear or quarrelling. Fear is the mentality of one who anticipates defeat. The battle is lost before it begins. Quarreling or fighting is to be unaware of happiness. Accordingly, victory is always followed by defeat. No one can win forever. Victory is the beginning of defeat in this world.

Kodokan judo, if considered as a piece of architecture, is a magnificent construction. Compared to that, aikido, of which I will speak later in this book, is the substructure of judo. It is the *do* (*tao*) itself. Aikido is a bridge leading to the *do* of judo.

I am not a master of the physical practice of judo. However, I have wholeheartedly and intensively researched physiological, psychological, and ideological judo. Each person is more or less gifted in certain areas. At any place and time each person has his or her own calling. A tenth degree master of Kodokan judo or even a master like Mr. Kano, the founder himself, cannot readily or easily explain the *do*. In our everyday life, the *do* (way of life) is much more applicable than the techniques of judo. If, through advanced age or sickness, it should become impossible for you to reach a high level in judo, you can still study and gain insight into the *do* and how to apply it to your everyday life. Grasping a concept through actual training is long and difficult; another way to grasp it is by thinking in terms of the words used to describe the underlying principles of its origin. This is direct, instantaneous, and intuitive.

Through understanding the way of life, the *do*, you will be able to strengthen the essence of your physical and ideological constitution and become a building block for the unification of all people in peace and freedom.

Chapter 1

A Tiny Pebble

Here is a tiny pebble that weighs half an ounce. If it falls from a height of one meter, it will have no noticeable effect whatsoever. If, however, it is dropped from a height of one thousand meters, various kinds of destruction may occur. It could possibly even take someone's life. This would depend on the speed of its fall or the ratio between distance and time. The shorter the time it takes to travel a given distance, the greater the power of the impact. According to modern science, the fastest speed on earth is the speed of light (186 thousand miles per second). This is the power used in the atomic bomb, which the whole world fears. Just imagine if we were able to harness the power of infinite speed. Regardless of how powerful our enemies or how insignificant our weapons, we could easily defeat them. Our weapons would be invincible. The reality of the situation is, however, that all of us in our everyday life observe this infinite energy in our thought and imagination. We are, in fact, using it all the time. We are able to instantaneously run through time and space regardless of the distance. We are even able to go in all directions simultaneously.

The ideal of aikido is to frecly use the infinite itself; to utilize the infinite speed energy of the benevolent love that embraces all things. This is the ultimate goal (*gokui*) of aikido. This kind of metaphorical or abstract explanation may be difficult to grasp so I will try to elaborate further.

"Everyone is happy; if not, it is their own fault," says Epictetus. I agree completely with this. I would go further to say that unhappy people are all criminals, including those who suffer from poverty, sickness, war, accident, germs, bacteria, oppression from others, and anxiety. I also include as criminals those who do not know what happiness and unhappiness are, what the self is, what nature is, what the world is, or the driving mechanism that causes the world and the universe to turn. In short, unhappy people are those who are afraid and do not know how to live without depending on some great outside power. Those who are unable to realize their dreams, to any extent and without any outside assistance, are unhappy. Unhappiness is not limited only to those who believe themselves to be so; those who believe that they are happy as well, if they cannot continually bear witness to it through the proof of their own lives, are also unhappy. Sooner or later and almost inevitably they also are visited by misfortune and go into a confused state of panic. Sometimes the ingredients of unhappiness have been building up slowly over a long period of time and have only gone undetected. By the time they realize it, they are already deeply immersed in misery and chaos. Unhappiness may seem like a typhoon that blows in and out again so quickly that there is happiness within unhappiness. This is our great chance to change ourselves and be forever saved from unhappiness. If we are so dull and complacent, however, that we can't even sense our own unhappiness, this chance will pass us by. The reason for this is that we become accustomed to the state of unhappiness and think it to be the normal state of human existence.

For example, let us imagine a young man. He is seemingly healthy and strong and is wealthy as well. He believes himself to be quite happy. Suppose he is killed in an accident. It is no one else's fault but his own. His extrasensory perception, or his instinct, is veiled. He is suffering from an illness that has caused a functional paralysis of his function of adaptability. This could be verified by autopsy at the time of the accident.

For a master of aikido or judo to die in an accident, or by sickness before the age of seventy, is unlikely. This person's physical, physiological, spiritual, sociological, and biological adaptability is healthy and strong. A true master would be able to avoid such an accident before it even occurred.

Judo and aikido nurture and develop adaptability to the highest degree. If such a master, therefore, could not be protected against a physical or physiological accident, how could this person even hope to resist the weapon of death invented by humanity? How could this person be protected against a sudden attack by someone with murderous intention? Adaptability, incidentally, is based on powers of memory and creative imagination—a kind of ability to foresee the future. If one is to become a master (*shihan*) of judo or aikido, one must be able to know beforehand all the various possibilities that might occur within time and space.

Omou and Kangaeru: Two Kinds of Thought

There are two kinds of totally contradictory memory and imagination or thought.

1. One kind of thought is of this relative world—transient, easily lost, and individual; for example: money, beauty, comfort, power, authority, jewels, food and drink, clothes, and personal rights.

2. Another kind of thought is that concerned with the eternal, infinite, absolute, unlimited world; for example: freedom, justice, peace, and truth. These are all unlimited, universal, unique, and very few in number.

Strangely enough, if you are able to clearly define any one of the items in the second category you will be able to obtain or create as much of any of the items in the first category as you like. Discover truth first, and it will liberate you.

In Japanese, the thinking function is expressed by two words. One is *omou,* and the other is *kangaeru.* These express the difference between the two different kinds of creative imagination. *Omou* is something like weighing the relative value of something through one's own mentality. *Kangaeru* means to return to God. Kangaeru is like prayer or meditation. 'Prayer' is probably closest to the correct meaning.

The adaptability that one gains through the practice of judo or aikido is similar to the idea of *kangaeru.* It is based on creative imagination and memory. Imagination and memory, or, in other words, prayer or meditation, are an intuitive perception of the world. They are like a minute and ultrasensitive compass that indicates immediately and automatically the direction we must take in order to practically accomplish utopia, or heaven on earth.

When we make the principle of Far Eastern science and philosophy a part of our physical being, this yin and yang compass begins to operate like a precision instrument. The philosophy of the Far East is the order and even the very structure of the universe. It is a practical dialectic as useful for daily cooking as for theoretical analysis of the ultimate construction of the atom. Confusion, disorder, and antagonism are the characteristics of our time. These contradictions and antagonisms are only one-ten-thousandth part of all the misunderstandings created through the undefined and indiscriminate use of words with double or contradictory (i.e., finite or relative and infinite or absolute) meanings. If you could discover the definitions for the most important words of the second kind of thought, one or two dozen at most, you would be able to solve almost any problem all by yourself. It would become possible to clarify confusion and end the most bitter conflicts without the need for killing endless numbers of innocent people and destroying both cultural and ideological constructions. If we could discover, for example, the meaning of the word 'justice,' it would have considerable impact. (See the list in Chapter 8, The Compass of Happiness.)

And yet, how is it possible for us to translate meditation, the power of imagination or prayer, into manifest realities here and now? This is accomplished through the intermediary of our millions of brain cells. Our brain is like a kind of radio receiver; through our invisible antennae of instinct, we receive signals from, and are put in touch with, the minds and actions of other people as well as animals. This includes the vibrations of all that occurs throughout this universal space-time continuum.

Accordingly, all of existence, from the tiniest imaginary electron to our huge solar system, is either the electromagnetic waves transmitted by all things or the bodies where those chaotic vibrations are brought together in an orderly fashion. This is an about-face of our thinking in the manner of Copernicus. Neither memory nor imagination nor thought are confined within our body; they are received from the outside. All of the great geniuses of all ages—Napoleon, Alexander the Great, Tutankhamen, Jesus, Buddha, Socrates, Plato, Genghis Khan, or Bach, Beethoven, Wagner, Marx, Cecil Rhodes, and Lesseps—were people in possession of the highest capacity receivers. They are all the translators, the revisers, and the editors of the various parts of even more ancient ideas. All of these great men were, through that which they had received, men of deep, wide, passionate, and powerful personality and character. This great power was, and is and always will be, of the same infinitely universal origin.

It is the brain, then, with its millions of cells that takes those universal vibrations and gathers them together and rearranges them in a new pattern. It filters them and produces a new idea. Differences in human personality are the result of physical, physiological, and biological differences.

The brain transfers an idea from the infinite memory (the main flow of the function of consciousness) into a concrete manifest reality; the change from ultrasensibility to physical, physiological, manifest sensibility, from thought to action. By words or performance, for example, forcing the majority of the audience into self-reflection, making them cry or become excited or experience some spiritual awakening such as in the case of a sermon given by a priest... all of this is accomplished without the use of any instrument or physical force.

Emerson said that the greatest thing we can accomplish in this world is to cause people to change their thinking, their actions, and become excited about accomplishing a great dream, to cause them to sacrifice everything for this dream.

Anyone who would ridicule these words doesn't understand the power of words or the great importance of the mechanism of thought or weeping. This person cannot make such a great discovery as Goethe made. Goethe spent his time from youth onward engrossed in thought and at last, in his later years, he was amazed to finally grasp the mysterious mechanism behind the processes of meditation, imagination, and thought itself. If you read Emerson's words and feel nothing, this is the real tragedy.

You may think, and rightly so, that all of this is quite bold. Indeed it is! It is a revolutionary way of thinking that dates back many thousands of years in the Far East. It belongs to the category of what Lévy-Bruhl called "primitive mentality," and it has never before been spread to the West. It is quite foreign in modern times, even to orientals themselves and, especially, to the westernized Japanese. I hope to explain it little by little in this book.

Like a tiny pebble that falls from a distant corner of the empty sky of infinity, I, a small existence without renown, hope to succeed in making the importance of these basic truths understood. If I can succeed in this, I will be very happy.

Chapter 2

Unifying East and West

Eugen Herrigel was a young German professor who spent some years in Japan and taught philosophy at Tokyo University between the wars. He was an expert with both a rifle and a pistol. In order to improve his understanding of Eastern philosophy, he decided to study some form of traditional martial or fine art. He chose archery.[5]

Archery, of course, exists also in the West and yet it is fundamentally quite different from Japanese *kyudo*. Herrigel decided to study *kyudo*. Japanese archery, like judo and aikido, is not to be classified among sports. *Kyudo* is a philosophy and also a formal religious ritual.

The young Herrigel was introduced to K. Awa *shihan*, a very typical Japanese master. The master, however, flatly refused to accept him as a student.

In Germany, Herrigel had tutored a Japanese student in German for three years. Thus, he was not altogether unfamiliar with the primitive mentality and the kind, childlike innocence of Japanese people. Regardless of repeated refusals, he tenaciously and patiently refused to give up his intention. Finally, with the recommendation of one of the master's students who was a teacher at Tohoku University in the same field as Herrigel, his wish was granted, and he was accepted as a student of Awa's.

However, the master only allowed him to perform the rudimentary basics for the first four to five years. That is, he practiced bowing and shooting arrows at large straw targets from a distance of two meters, an exceedingly boring practice for anyone. This was all the more difficult for Herrigel, a master target shooter with a pistol, to endure.

One day in his fifth year of study, which was toward the end of his stay in Japan, at about nine in the evening, he was summoned by the master. As with all masters of *budo* and also the traditional Japanese fine arts (*geido*), master Awa spoke no German and seldom spoke at length even in his own language. The master took his young Western student and his wife to the *kyudo dojo*. As it was night, it was impossible to see the target, which was sixty meters distant. The master then lit a tiny piece of incense and placed it in front of the target. At sixty meters, the tiny light from the incense was almost impossible to see. The master then shot two arrows into the night and asked Herrigel to retrieve them. The first arrow rested in the bull's eye, and the second one had split the first. When Herrigel saw this, he was stunned with amazement. *Kyudo* is definitely not a sport! In the eyes of beginners, it can be seen only as magic or a kind of mystical technique. At last, this meaning sank deeply into Herrigel's consciousness. At the same time, he understood why it was impossible for him to learn much in five years. He had been too full of confidence in himself and his own art. He thought he could grasp the unknown Japan in a Western fashion. Instead of learning Japanese culture or thinking, he had tended to criticize or judge according to his own knowledge or standards. It seems that he had expected to understand Japan in the image of his own country or that of the West in general. Beyond this, he was not able to comprehend, not within the first five years.

Japan is another world entirely. It may be called a society of the primitive mind. *Kyudo* (the way of the bow) and the pistol master, or in other words Japan and the Western world, are exactly like two ends of a magnet. The North views the direction of the South as mistaken while the South, for its part, probably feels that it is the North that is going in the wrong direction.

East is East and West is West and never the twain shall meet—so stated Kipling. This is a large oversight. It is not true at all. It shows a very limited understanding. Yes, of course, East is East and West is West, but aren't these only two different names for one and the same earth? That is to say, they are neither the same nor are they different.

The East exists within the West, and the West exists within the East. From a relative point of view, their differences emerge, and yet they are the same in an absolute sense. The logic of Aristotle and Kant is not applicable here.

If East and West set out to injure each other and refuse to recognize the connection between them, they will both end in genocide. However, East and West are complementary. For either to understand their own nature, they will have to know their complementary partner. They must know the dialectic constitution and structure of the earth, the world, and the universe. East cannot exist without West and vice versa.

The Far East seems to be a world of primitive and backward mentality to Westerners. To Orientals, on the other hand, Western society appears altogether foolish and infantile. They must try to understand each other, and they can if they really have the sincere intention and desire to do so. If they lead each other toward a society of mutual honor, appreciation, and respect and really grasp the order of the universe, it will very easily be accomplished.

Americans have the tendency to treat each other with a great deal of politeness. If both East and West were to take up such a civil manner in relationships with all outside countries, the need for national boundaries would be eliminated and there would be no further recurrence of war.

After five years, young professor Herrigel discovered the nature and mentality of the Far East. Basic and simple things require the greatest effort to grasp. Ah, if only Herrigel had realized the greatness of Eastern mind and spirit when he first arrived. If only he had been a little more physically flexible, with a firmer will and determination. The problem is arrogance and fear. In the first place, the real problem is the attitude of cynicism and exclusivity that exists between different races. It is this which draws all people into conflict. It is the most difficult problem to cure.

No one is perfect. There is good and bad within all, both East and West. But if people are able to really feel a sense of internationalism and make the order of the universe an integral part of their own being, real understanding between people will become possible and they can discover their mutual strengths as well as deficiencies.

If America had taken one-ten-thousandth of the money that was spent on World War II and donated it towards research on primitive mentality, after the fashion of Professor Lévy-Bruhl, or if they had, without spending even a penny, aided certain Japanese laborers who wanted to emigrate to South America during the war, they would have saved an enormous amount of money and countless human lives. Above and beyond the saving of precious time, they would have also gained great respect and admiration.

Certainly the foolish behavior of Japan's modern-day samurai was unprecedented in Japanese history, and yet America could have been honored as a guardian and organizer of world peace rather than merely gaining a victory of bloodshed.

Of course, not America alone is to be criticized. The Japanese themselves could not then, nor can they now, recognize the greatness of their own primitive mentality. This is all the more reason why they are unable to grasp that which is great in Western society. In spite of this, they have continued right up to the present to Westernize themselves as quickly as possible. This spiritual self-colonization is wretched and pitiful. It completely undermines the foundations of mutual international understanding. It is somewhat understandable if the crow wishes to adorn himself with the peacock's feathers, but is there a peacock who wrenches off his beautiful feathers hoping to wear those of the crow?

Such advanced adaptability (as is witnessed in the techniques of judo, *kyudo*, and aikido) is, on first exposure, quite incomprehensible to the Western mentality, which has been raised with a completely opposite set of sensibilities. Japanese archery is not an art for fighting or for killing one's enemies. Quite the contrary. It is the way of making the marksman become the bow and arrow and the bow and arrow become the marksman's will. In other words, it is a method of unifying the marksman, the bow and arrow, the practice hall, and the infinite universe into one body by eliminating one's usual dependence on the five senses.

This is completely different from Western society or almost all other schools of thought, including those of scientists, scholars, or those who believe in the laws and moral codes passed down by traditional religion. All people are born with the protective mechanism of instinctive and intuitive ability. This is especially apparent in small children and animals. The formidable opponent, which gradually kills the instinct and intuition that we carry with us from birth, is modern education.

Could it have been primitive people who invented such abominable tools of destruction as the atomic bomb that was dropped on the developing country of Japan? Decidedly not. Adaptability is first of all the function that allows us to protect and preserve ourselves under the various pressures of intimidation and the ultimate threat of our own death or extinction. It is the composite of our powers of memory, judgment, thought, and will. Among these various aspects, however, memory is the mother of reasoning, judgment, thought, choice, and intuition. It is the source of our instinct itself.

All scholarly knowledge, as well as our everyday knowledge, is the composite of our sense data that has been compiled in our mind, polished, refined, analyzed, put into order, recognized, and remembered. This is equally true for both the natural and the cultural (human) sciences. From the moment the sperm takes residence in the ovule, memory is the single most important factor in our life. Our very first cell, our microscopic embryological seed, has already secured a marvelous adaptability. It knows very well those things it must take and those it must not. In a word, our embryological seed has the ability to choose. It is, in fact, an analysis specialist. Floating within the torrential sea of nutritious elements, this tiny seed instantaneously and without the use of any instrument analyzes them all. It is this unit of memory and judgment that creates our entire personality and constitution.

If you were able to control your memory at will, what fantastic things you could accomplish. All true schools of the *do* promote, polish, refine, and strengthen this innate faculty of memory. Memory is the basic construction that unifies our life energy itself. All people who reach some degree of mastery of the *do*, even though their lifestyles and professions may be different, have a remarkable ability to understand each other. The memories of even the lesser students, who are unable to receive the higher certificates of accomplishment of *do*, are not dulled like those who graduate from Western schools. These students still have the appropriate qualities for becoming good citizens of a free society. All the evils of humanity result from the decline, decay, and sickness of the memory. In contrast, all of the virtues of humanity originate from ample, healthy memory and bright, unveiled instinct.

All of the inventions born from Western philosophical, technical, scientific, and religious education that are not backed up by an intuitive comprehension of the world and the universe are extremely dangerous. The techniques that one learns intuitively in any school of the *do* are the key to setting foot on the immense, and as yet unknown, continent of human possibility. The function of ESP (extrasensory perception), researched at Duke University, is the doorway to the infinite and incredible possibilities of memory. Yet, thanks to modern education, that door has all but completely been closed again. The way of the *do*, however, stands open for all who are sincere and pure of heart. Western education has, since the time of the Renaissance, Copernicus, Galileo, and Da Vinci, gradually taken advantage of the decline of the traditional Eastern teachings imported by Jesus, Democritus, and Heraclitus, the great masters of the *do*. Everything that has a beginning has an end.

Western education began at a particular time and, therefore, must also end. The *do*, however, is just like the primitive mind. It has neither beginning nor end. If the Eastern schools of Christianity, Buddhism, and Taoism could not escape this law, it is because their founders, being mortal, can hardly escape, one by one, meeting their untimely deaths. All of the Western schools, whether in natural or cultural science or the sciences of biology and medicine, are all aimed at and are all progressing toward their end. Western education lacks the uniform rules that will judge, lead, and control all philosophies, all scientific knowledge and technique. That is to say, there is no Western technique or science that is founded on the unifying principle of yin and yang. The main characteristics of Western education are professionalism and fractionalization, both of which stand in opposition to an understanding of the unique principle of the *do* (the way of life according to nature's laws and the order of the universe). They lack the axial compass of a practical dialectic, a universal worldview, an understanding of the order of the universe. Accordingly, there is an absolute and urgent necessity to create a new, unifying culture based on the *tao* (*do*), like that of the Far East.

The East and the West are both standing at the same starting point. The one who first realizes this and applies it will be the greatest benefactor of humanity not only in the twentieth century but for all time.

Chapter 3

Seeds of Conflict

Two children, five years old, have a fight or quarrel. They have no weapons whatsoever. They are unaware that such things even exist. When they reach the age of ten or twelve, they may use sticks or stones to fight with. This is the beginning of military arms. Furthermore, as the years go by and they become adults, their mentality becomes more fixed and confined to certain limitations. They begin to self-reflect. When there is a difference of opinion among them, they discuss it openly or by letter, utilizing intellect and reasoning. They are acutely aware of the fact that forceful confrontation serves no purpose whatsoever. This is instinctive and universal. It is based on reason and rationality. In any case, they avoid bloody confrontation and seek to prohibit it at all costs. They strive to prohibit the use of weapons, which can kill one another.

Let us review some points of human history. Some hundreds of thousands of years ago, in the infancy of the human race, people fought amongst themselves using their hands, teeth, and nails. Toward the end of that period, they began to use fire, the sword, and bows and arrows. Still, thousands of years later, as we enter into the age of humankind's youth, a new weapon, one which prohibits the use of all murderous weapons, came into being. This new weapon was law. It was a miraculous breakthrough for the human race: the victory of human reason and instinct over easily unstable passion and emotion. This is a point in human progress worthy of notice. It is, in fact, the seed of culture and civilization.

The Ferments of War

Humankind, however, has entered into the most huge, disgusting, cowardly, and foolish conflict on the stage of humanity and social intercourse. This is war or international conflict. It is a new kind of conflict involving two or more countries. It is completely different from a quarrel between two individuals. There are four indispensable elements for war:

• A very strong dictator, group of leaders, or government guided by a wrong worldview. They will say that it is the idea of the representatives elected by the people, but, in actuality, the people are misled by the power of a small political faction or party, imposing itself like an unwanted dictator. Under the name of law, the people are intimidated and led into war by undesirable dictators, political parties, and the government. Regardless of whether it is one political party or many, unless they are impartially guided by a very sensitive and ultra-accurate compass, we cannot say that their way is correct.

• A people without a world concept who, in the face of intimidation by a powerful adversary, will readily and willingly comply with any and all demands in order to protect themselves.

• Constant progress and advancement in creating ever more terrifying and atrocious weapons to fortify a government or dictator.

• Finally, fear is the piston or greatest driving force perpetuating a false conception of the world. Fear is hidden under the guise of attack or ambition to secure, through trickery or brute force, the kind of shelter, weapons, or authority through which one can be assured of one's own safety. In order to protect personal interests, profits, and territory at all costs, governments and dictators are led by fear to intentionally or unintentionally sacrifice the lives of countless human beings. Fear is actually the driving force that throws people into the quagmire of war. Weapons and artillery are only symbols of that fear. The more powerful the weapons, the greater is the fear on the part of those who require and depend upon them. Furthermore, fear is nothing more than one physiological expression of those who cannot perceive a universal worldview of life and reality.

Thus, the ultimate cause of war is a combination of three factors: fear and uneasiness that necessitate the creation of more and more powerful weapons; governments and dictators who control these weapons and the law in whatever way they please; and egotistical people who think only of their own profits and, due to ignorance, believe that the violence known as majority rule is the highest virtue. These three factors, united by the catalyst of fear, begin to ferment, react, and respond to each other. This eventually changes into a state of chaos and confusion and, upon making contact with another similarly fermenting situation, unleashes the violent reaction of war.

To reiterate, war is the blind desire for a comfortable life, two countries both desiring to monopolize all natural resources for themselves. This can lead to the end of material civilization and culture. It is a kind of sickness or insanity. Turning toward his children, a man teaches them not to take life or to quarrel with others. Then turning around, he plunges himself headlong into a brutal and cold-blooded war. When mental disease reaches this point, it is a very grave psychosis.

The only cure for this sickness is an understanding of the unique principle of the order of the universe. The only way to solve the problem of modern confusion and unrest is to give birth to a new state modeled after this natural order. We must realize that a state cannot survive by force alone. The problem is, however, what can we do to actually realize this? It is self evident that war cannot be eradicated by force. Stopping war with force is like trying to put out a fire with fire. This is not possible without sacrificing everything. It would be the suicide of humanity. But, it is not so simple a thing as putting out a fire; for this we only need to use the opposite of fire. The opposite of force is reason. Reason encompasses and judges all things. This is the very principle of judo. This principle itself is a unique, unparalleled, universal worldview. It is a compass that points out a new direction towards eternal peace and freedom.

But I suppose you will raise your voice to object, saying that humans have more than enough rationality already. The type of reason of which I am speaking here is not the same as that which underlies today's modern civilization. It is not the kind of reason spoken of by Gandhi. The reason of which I speak encompasses the entire universe. I speak of a reasoning power that can create the technical ability to bring people to live in peace and freedom. This reasoning power or intuitive judgment is a sensitive and precise compass that leads humanity toward happiness. It is the reason or principle of the order of the universe itself that allows people to realize their happiness anytime or anyplace and to accomplish all that they dream or desire without the need for any particular tool or implement.

The religion of Jesus Christ was one example of this kind of reason. The Christianity of today is, however, a false interpretation of that example. It is a fragmented fossil of it. The same is true in the case of Confucius. There is a great deal of exclusivity in both Christianity and Confucianism. A truly universal view must include everything. There can be no exclusion or exception. It is a reason that judges, comprehends, and embraces all things.

This kind of reason is called the *tao* (*do*), the way. Judo is the flexible or soft way of self-defense. Others are *chado*, the way of tea; *kendo*, the way of the sword; *shodo*, the way of calligraphy; *kado*, the way of flowers; and *ido*, the way of medicine. All the traditional paths of study passed down from ancient times are based on the *do*, as is shown by their respective names. These are all different paths toward one and the same end. In a word, they all aim at grasping the key to the kingdom of heaven, the order of the universe.

Western System of Combat

Why in the world is it, then, that we make war? From 1940 to 1945 we carried on, at enormous cost, a great war which was to end war for all time.

- More than 32 million young men in the prime of their lives were killed on the battlefield.
- Between 15 and 20 million women, children, and elderly people were killed in air raids.

- 26 million people were assassinated in concentration camps.
- 29 million people became wanderers, mutilated or otherwise incapacitated for productive work.
- 21 million people lost their homes and all fortune or possessions due to bombings.
- 45 million people became refugees or separated from their homes by thousands of miles.
- 30 million homes were reduced to ashes.
- 150 million people were left homeless and suffering from famine and illness
- One million children were left orphans and one million parents lost their children.
- Between 45 and 50 million were left with no jobs, no family, nothing.

World War II (1940-1945) cost three times more than World War I (1914-1918); that is, 375 billion dollars. With this amount of money one could buy a splendid house and furnishings for every family of the United States, Canada, Russia, Australia, England, Ireland, France, and Belgium, and still have enough left over to give each family a present of $200,000. To each city of 200,000 or more inhabitants, one could make a donation of $10 million for libraries, $10 million for schools, and the same to build hospitals. These figures tell the whole story.

The above is the cost of World War II. With this amount of money, we could give $400,000 to every family on the earth. Nevertheless, the species of the animal kingdom that calls itself the spiritual leader of all nature's creations left a great blemish on its own history by dropping the first two atomic bombs and killing 313,814 of its own kind.

Among those killed were thousands of women and children, nursing babies, sick and bedridden people, as well as honest hardworking laborers. Hospitals and schools were demolished instantaneously. The War ended with the unconditional surrender of Japan and yet, by 1950, another fifteen wars had already taken place. This fire of war is still smoldering.

In a message addressed to American mothers, Mrs. Eleanor Roosevelt declared, "Since the end of the War, there has not ceased to be fighting in some corner of the world." Franklin D. Roosevelt's widow was mistaken on only one point: fighting had gone on not only in one place or another but in many places simultaneously. Actually, we have put certain small incidents out of mind. Japan surrendered on September 2, 1945. The same day, about six hours later, the armies of Mao Tse-tung launched their first offensive in Northern China. One month later, October 1945, marked the beginning of the civil war in Greece. And then, from that time:

- 1945 war in Lebanon; bombardment of Damascus; civil war in Malaysia.
- 1946 civil war in Burma; beginning of war (November) in Indochina; revolt of the Hukse (Philippines).
- 1947 (May 29) revolt in Madagascar; (July 20) war in Indonesia; (July) riot in Punjab.
- 1948 (May 15) war of Palestine; India against Pakistan; war of Hyderabad, India; civil war in Yemen (for the succession of the king); 1950, the Korean War.

There were continual wars and bloodshed, including border incidents that were very deadly, and also the "white" wars between England and Yemen after 1947, where the shooting was mostly in the air and little damage was done. The riots of the Punjab, on the contrary, which didn't receive much attention, took in only three years no less than several million victims.

Humankind has made such tremendous progress both theoretically and in the invention of countless things. Why is it then that among many nations there is the constant recurrence of such bloody and destructive wars? The value of life is well known to all, and yet the utmost is done to destroy it. If this isn't madness, what is?

Moreover, victories won by great force are never lasting. Victories gained in modern warfare are the same as defeat. Spending enormous amounts of money in order to kill each other is the height of stupidity. When the maxim "time is money" first came to Japan from America, it caused quite a stir. We felt a mixture of curiosity and sorrow. The time of our life is so short as to be insufficient compared to the eternal time of the universe. To us, time is far too precious a thing to compare with money. If, however, such a maxim can be accepted in the West, how then is it possible for America and Europe to engage in war where both time and money are carelessly thrown away? It is completely distressing to try to comprehend this absurd behavior of human beings. There is no other animal that displays this amount of stupidity. Even the meager existence of a simple flea makes no attempt to imitate such foolishness.

Battles of Early Japan

In ancient times, there was a small country with a mysterious name, "the macrobiotic country of the far eastern seas where people know the secret of eternal youth, long life, and how to live in freedom and happiness." This was more than two thousand years ago, 215 years before the time of Christ. At that time, Shin, the first emperor of the world kingdom of China, dispatched a special envoy to this country in the eastern seas, which was also known as the Land of the Rising Sun (Japan). Their purpose was to study and research the science and philosophy of this small macrobiotic country. It was, at that time, the country of the samurai.

Samurai translates into Western language as soldier or warrior, but in fact its true meaning is quite different. Another name given to the samurai was *mono no fu*, which means a free man who intuitively understands the meaning of nature, society, and the universe. He is a philosopher who has grasped the reality of the world, a poet who composed poems on the battlefield in either Japanese or classic Chinese. He relates to all of life and the environment in terms of nature and the order of the universe and paints pictures of his own impressions.

He was not merely a soldier, a warrior, or a man of power. The meaning of his life was quite different. This warrior, artist, and poet was always prepared to solve any unexpected difficulties that might arise in the moment. Of course, such a warrior was the ideal and somewhat rare. Yet among the great samurai, there were none without these qualities. The land of the samurai was, in fact, so agreeable that the emissaries of the first emperor of China stayed there for the rest of their natural lives rather than return to their own country. They preferred not to return to their homeland, which was under dictatorial rule.

Some reading of the *Manyoshu*,[6] which was compiled in the Nara period (eighth century), will suffice to discover hundreds of samurai-poets who composed poems far more profound and philosophical than many of those written today.

Of course, in the Land of the Rising Sun, there were also battles from time to time. Yet these cannot be compared with the wars of the West. The battles of early Japan were examples of great courage, decorum, and manners, even elegance and refinement. I will present a few examples.

The year was around 919 A.D. in the province of Musashi (present-day Tokyo). There were two great samurai generals, Yuzuru Minamoto and Yoshibumi Taira.[7] They had been quarrelling with each other for a very long time. One day Yuzuru sent one of his samurai bearing a letter for Yoshibumi. It was written in a formal style after the custom of generals, but an abbreviated summary would be like this: I would like to propose a method of bringing our long feud to a satisfactory conclusion. If you find these terms agreeable, I would be extremely grateful. The two of us—you, Lord Yoshibumi of Taira, and I, Yuzuru of Minamoto, without any tricks and in the full presence of our armies—shall openly vie with each other. If I should be defeated, you may take all that belongs to me. If, on the other hand, I should be victorious, I will receive all that is yours.

The response to this letter was none other than enthusiastic agreement. At the appointed hour, the two generals approached each other on horseback and commenced fighting. The battle lasted for hours.

At first, they rode back and forth, shooting arrows at each other. When their supply of arrows was exhausted, they began to duel with swords. Suddenly, the long sword of Minamoto was broken. With this, Taira also tossed his own sword onto the ground, and they began a fierce battle of full body contact. This tremendous battle continued for a long time until finally Minamoto cried out in a loud voice, "My Lord, I now understand that there is no difference in our ability and power. Regardless of how long we continue, there will be no end to this battle. It will go on for hours and then for days. Because it is useless, let us call an end to it and establish peace and friendship. Let us combine our forces together."

This proposal was accepted with great pleasure and everyone, after seeing the fierce battle of their leaders, was completely satisfied. There was not one complaint from either side. From that time on, understanding and friendly relations were established. It is said that this cooperation lasted even after the death of these great leaders.

In the sixteenth century too, there were some great samurai generals who were also philosophers and poets. Among these, the most famous were Shingen Takeda and Kenshin Uesugi. A battle between these two great generals continued for more than ten years (1551-1564). Takeda's territory was in the mountains far from the sea. It was a small country like Switzerland and was called "the country of Kai." The people of Kai suffered from a lack of salt, and it was none other than Kenshin Uesugi who, from time to time, furnished them with it.

Finally, at last, in 1564 the curtain fell on the most famous war in Japanese history. One day in August, Takeda sent one of his samurai, Hikoroku Yasuba, with a letter for his enemy, General Kenshin Uesugi: "It is with great joy that I suggest to you a method of bringing our long and drawn-out war to an end. Our people have long suffered and been distressed by this war. We must relieve them of this suffering. I, therefore, suggest that we hold an individual combat between the two strongest warriors of our respective armies."

Kenshin accepted this proposal and fixed the day and the hour of the combat —August 11, 1564. The warrior representing Shingen's army was Hikoroku Yasuba. He was a huge man astride a large horse.

Representing Kenshin was Kiren Hasebe, a man of small stature and riding a small horse. The two fought for many hours, and finally Hasebe got the upper hand, pinned his opponent to the ground, and beheaded him. Then, in the ancient custom of the samurai, Hasebe raised the head in his left hand and declared his name and his victory: "For all those present, I, Kiren Hasebe, the servant of the Lord Kenshin Uesugi, humbly announce to Lord Shingen Takeda that I have, in his presence, beheaded the representative of his army, Hikoroku Yasuba." In this way, justice was achieved without the destruction of property or large numbers of people.

Takeda transferred ownership of the four most important territories in his possession over to General Uesugi, and they remained very close friends from that time on. Six years later, Takeda passed away. Upon hearing of his death, Kenshin was so filled with grief that he could not eat at all for some time. This episode is well known. Kenshin Uesugi was a great political and economic reformer. He reorganized, in accordance with the order of the universe, the way of life of his people who had until that time led miserable and wretched lives. His martial regiments, as well as his literary educational programs, were splendid achievements. Even today, the people of Kenshin's district are distinguished and respectable. They are known for their sobriety, patience, and strong will. The social organization and the educational system established by this samurai-philosopher-poet have lasted over 400 years. It is truly wonderful. Today, the people of Japan hold Kenshin in great respect, love, and admiration.

In order to save millions of lives and billions of dollars, why don't Truman and Stalin hold a duel between themselves alone? It would be much more civilized if they would hold the battle on the borderline of their respective territories in Eastern Siberia and fight naked without weapons, in the style of the Olympics. If someone would begin to sell reserved-seat tickets immediately, billions of dollars could be made.

Chapter 4

Judo and the Unique Principle

Why did human beings begin such a cruel, costly, and dangerous practice as war? The answer is quite simple. It is because they do not know the principles of an art such as judo. Or, we can say, it is because their memory and imagination, these being the factors that activate reason and good-naturedness, are sick and weak. It is the lenticular cataract of humanity. Completely unknown in the West, there is in the Far East a wonderful medicine for this sickness. It is about this that I would like to speak in this chapter.

If, however, you suffer from the very same illness, or if you have been unable to comprehend or remember what you have read so far; if you don't know even one way to stop the cruel and useless practice of war that you detest so much, if you do not live each day with great joy, or if you do not find pleasure in reading the words of Epictetus, "Everyone is happy; if not, it is their own fault," then you must first read and understand the following chapters on the new method of macrobiotics, a practical physiology that includes Eastern philosophy and science. Then you must, for at least a week, very carefully put all that you have read into practice.

If you didn't have any memory, you would be unable to read this book at all. This is not a novel for merely passing the time away or a book for passing along factual knowledge. What I am endeavoring to accomplish with this book is to present a new method through which all people, at any time or place, can live in unending happiness. I am attempting to supply you with the key to the kingdom of heaven. This is not merely a book for the purpose of explaining the techniques of judo.

The origin of judo precedes recorded history. It is a philosophy, a school of aesthetics, a theory, and an actual practice all in one. As I have already mentioned, judo is a highly developed and refined expression of our instinctive adaptability. It is nothing other than the intrinsic nature of instinct, which is, in turn, the fountainhead of life energy and consciousness itself. In this sense, we can understand the origin of judo as instinct. How, when, and where, depending on some particular individual, the technical practice of judo began is a question that is not under examination here.

The first problem in judo is that of power. Judo is a fine art of human energy. When judo is considered as a fine art, it really begins with the most economical use of physical power or strength. It is with this point that we find the difference between man and other animals. Animals use their physical power automatically, without considering method. An animal has never invented a lever.

Let us recall here the fact that force or power is the function of matter passing through space in a fixed period of time. The shorter the time, the greater the force.

The discovery of a straight pole as a weapon was quite an invention. It was the beginning of military arms. The idea of a stone-headed spear is an invention that did not come about without a great deal of pondering and mental effort. This was the first step toward modern firepower. Modern weapons utilize dynamics, in addition to the use of space, to be able to defend oneself at a distance. With this principle, little David was able to kill Goliath the giant. Even the atomic bomb is only a further extension of this principle, that is, to be able to kill the enemy from a distance without exposing oneself to attack.

However, venturing to attack from a distance under a shelter and with a weapon that is not in the possession of the enemy or which is superior to that of the enemy is regarded, in the country of the samurai, as the most detestable and cowardly conduct. Even today, this is forbidden in games and sports. The great majority of the countries of the world honor justice in sports. The spirit of impartiality and fair play has, on the other hand, been completely denied in the much more important and decisive practice of war. What is the reason for this? It is necessary to consider this problem well.

Forgetting the principles of judo for a moment, can we eliminate war through war, eradicate unreasonableness and brute force by the use of such force, which is totally lacking in principle? Are we to assume that sports determine the boundaries of the frontier of justice and that everything else is outside of this frontier? If this is the case, how is it then that we can hope to establish peace through war? Is it really possible to establish peace through the utilization of an unjust method? That which we wish to establish is peace depending on justice, is it not? To utilize the most detestable and cowardly means in order to annihilate the enemy at any cost is hardly honorable or commendable. It is borrowing the power of the devil. To destroy the enemy and buy a victory in this world by the assistance of the devil is to sell both justice and one's soul as well. This is much too costly a bargain. It is for this very reason that all victory in this life is so ephemeral.

"You know that it has been said, an eye for an eye and a tooth for a tooth, but I say unto you, do not resist evil treatment. Rather, if someone strikes you on the right cheek, turn to him the other one also." (Matthew 5:38-39)

"And to those who wish to dispute in judgment with you and remove your tunic from you, give up also your cloak." (Matthew 5:40)

The above is Jesus Christ's interpretation of the principle of judo. Unfortunately, however, no one knows how to practically apply this principle in everyday life. Either Jesus didn't teach this aspect or Matthew forgot to record that part of Jesus's teaching. Later, I will very simply explain this principle in such a way that anyone can practice it with great pleasure.

Not being aware of this principle, people have continued with this thinking—"an eye for an eye" and an atomic bomb for an atomic bomb—for the past two thousand years. Moreover, people continue desperately trying to invent a weapon more powerful than that of the enemy. What kind of punishment will we have to endure before we cease such madness? In any case, the question at hand is whether or not it is possible to correct this erroneous mentality.

Charles Lindbergh was a very courageous pilot and a true seeker of the original cause of evil, and yet he was satisfied with his observation that the distance of one meter of extra speed could be the deciding factor in a merciless air battle. Are America and the other countries of the world really interested in selling justice and their own souls to gain victory by the power of Satan? I don't think so. It is only that their instinct has become weak and sick.

In other words, due to physical illness, they have done considerable damage to their memory. It is in an enfeebled state. They are no longer able to draw on the events of the past for their source of judgment. When they read the Bible, they seem to understand its message, and they are emotionally moved by it. But a few minutes later, they are no longer able to recall what it was that had such a profound effect on them. Once a week, they recall the Bible's message to their minds, but their memories are on vacation, sleeping, during the other six days. This is a mental disease. This is schizophrenia. If not, then they are living an egotistical lie and suffering from spiritual nearsightedness. This is a serious defect of the physiological constitution, the cure for which I will explain later. One cannot attack or criticize another's constitution without showing the ultimate cause and means of reconstruction.

Let's return for now to the history of judo. The origin of judo is, of course, strength or physical power. Beginning from this point, one country of the Far East, or perhaps we should say some few leaders of that country, utilized every power in their means to research and seek out the most economical and morally acceptable method for putting an end to the cruel and dangerous practice of war. In the West, however, people of small wisdom, cowardice, and cunning minds were leaning towards a different direction altogether. They sought, through research, to fortify themselves with ever more powerful and cruel military weapons.

Eastern people, especially the elite, had already completed such research thousands of years prior. This kind of research is among the classic literature of the East and is known as the Seven Canons of Strategy. The original Eastern strategy of war has its origins in the three great religions of humanity, a world conception based on Far Eastern science and philosophy and the unique principle of the order of the universe. The research of the Western elite, however, chose the path of perfecting the ultimate weapon. Finally, they arrived at the most inhuman firepower yet discovered, the atomic bomb. And their research still continues.

However you look at it, East and West are ultimately of the same origin. They have the same starting point, that is, instinct. It is their course that has become completely opposite. Why have they become so different? Seeing this from the physiological, biological, and philosophical view, it is an extremely interesting problem. I will speak of it at the very end of this book.

In any case, a people who continue to research increasingly inhuman weapons must eventually become aware that the use of weapons and force for fighting is useless; the goal will never be reached. It is a vicious cycle. Those who do not depend on weapons at all but rather research justice, love, and the establishment of absolute and lasting peace and harmony quite naturally arrive at judo and the strategy of peace (the Seven Canons). The object of judo is not to kill or destroy the enemy by force. It is rather to give them exactly whatever they desire, to divide and separate their energy and then reconstruct it. By applying the appropriate technical dynamics, this can be accomplished physiologically and philosophically, and you can change your enemy into a good friend.

In about the year 1642, the forerunner of the first school of judo was established. A samurai named Jushin Sekiguchi established one kind of judo. Sekiguchi himself was a disciple of both the great sword master Yagyu and also the Buddhist philosopher Takuan. Properly speaking, what he created was a form of *jujitsu* (or *jujutsu*). Sekiguchi had compiled and improved upon techniques that had been developed over many centuries.

Towards the end of the nineteenth century, the art flourished and was in its prime. There were hundreds of schools of *jujitsu*. Then came the Meiji Restoration,[8] this marked the end of the feudal era, and all the institutions and past systems were overthrown. The samurai lost their lords and their exalted position as well. They no longer had money even for food. The ancient weapons of the sword and the spear were all replaced by the new and modern firearms, which the samurai so greatly detested. All the teachers of judo and *kendo* lost their students.

At that pivotal time a young professor, Jigoro Kano, was teaching political philosophy and logic at Tokyo University. In 1882, he established the Kodokan (literally, school of the *tao* (*do*) or the unique principle of the Far East) School of Judo. This was accomplished by uniting all the older dying and decaying schools of *jujitsu* and reassembling all of their respective masters under his new form.

When Kano was seventy years old, he discovered a totally new form of judo that was relatively unknown. It was *aikido*, a second branch from *jujitsu*, created by the great master Morihei Ueshiba. Aikido is the most perfected form of judo. He wanted to learn it at once but, unfortunately, he was already an old man, and the severe training necessary for the task was beyond him. He, therefore, did the next best thing. He sent one of his best disciples, Minoru Mochizuki, to the school of Master Ueshiba. Mochizuki studied with Ueshiba for twenty years; he reached the level of eighth *dan* (degree) and became one of Ueshiba's highest students. I will tell more of Kano and Ueshiba in chapters 5 and 6, respectively.

The Goal of Judo

My version of the history of judo is first and foremost philosophical, physiological, and biological. To summarize, it is the same as all the arts of combat and defense throughout the world. Judo walks steadily on the path towards justice and seeks everlasting peace and harmony. There are some very special techniques in judo, however, that distinguish it from other arts or sports. One example is the art of *katsu*, bringing people back to consciousness who pass out during practice, combat, or swimming. The teacher of judo also knows the art of setting bones or adjusting various parts of the body when someone is injured; the master of judo inevitably knows both osteology and anatomy. If this were not the case, how could one control and dominate an opponent larger and stronger than oneself?

Judo is something beyond mere technique. It is a kind of medicine, a philosophical and religious exercise. It could also be called a sport that incorporates religion. It is a practical application of philosophy and the dialectic principle of the universe. It is a physical representation and expression of the unique principle and the order of the universe. You may verify this by observing a great teacher of judo or either any of the schools of the *do*. They are all world federalists.[9] They live by the principles of peace, harmony, and freedom. True judo masters have no excess. They are flexible and usually of small physical stature. They forbid the use of judo outside of the *dojo* (practice hall) except in the case of emergency or danger. It is not an art of attack. In judo, an attitude of defiance is also forbidden. One must not turn away or hide when it becomes necessary to swallow one's pride.

As it states in the Bible, we must "turn the other cheek." This is not, however, a matter of conscious decision but, rather, a natural result of our training. It is not at all intolerable. Rather, it is seen as a practical application of the principle underlying judo technique. As such, it is received with both gratitude and interest. It can even be a deeply emotional experience that contributes to understanding and progress. When this feeling is translated into actual judo technique, it develops the kind of ability that allows one to withstand repeated blows without injury. Because of this ability, we also are able to learn that we really do not have even one enemy in this world. All people are our good friends. The difficulties that they present us with help us to understand our own physiological and philosophical defects. So-called enemies help us to refine and perfect our conception of reality and the dynamic laws governing the construction of universal order. This is, therefore, quite a bit more practical and interesting than any form of religion. It can change the weakest, most ignorant, most backward or seemingly primitive person into the strongest, most perceptive, most civilized, happy person.

The goal of judo is to provide the physical and physiological compass with which to show all people, regardless of age, sex, education, or race, the true direction and practical method towards harmony (happiness) and freedom (health). It is to give them the unique principle of life and to provide a practical means for understanding it both intellectually and intuitively. The goal of judo is to render the use of unreasonable force useless and to eliminate all evil, all conflicts, all war and disputes. This very much resembles the true medicine, the original *ido*, that desires to establish physiological, individual, and social peace and harmony. The person with this totally healthy state of body and mind has no need whatsoever for modern conventional medicine or all the various problems that surround it.

Because such a spirit did exist at one time (in spite of some civil wars of a completely different nature than Western war), both China and Japan enjoyed total peace and harmony for a long time. Unhappily, however, after the importation of Western civilization, the spirit of judo and the strategy of peace were rapidly expelled. Gresham's law[10] operates here. In much the same way as the plague or Genghis Khan once devastated Europe, the mechanical civilization of the West has also robbed the treasures of the way of life, the *do*, and has left the East in a state of chaos. Tagore, Romain Rolland,[11] and Tenshin Okakura[12] bitterly detested this and resisted it as much as possible. Nonetheless, herein lies the very uniqueness of the gentle way of the Far East. As written in an ancient proverb, everything and everyone is part of their divine mission, and they, therefore, accept everything with respect and gratitude. This magnanimity includes even the thief, the bandit, and the scheming, deceitful one of evil deeds. This is also the uniqueness of judo; judo is known as the soft or gentle martial art.

Upon arriving in Tokyo, MacArthur declared that to the extent the Japanese did not accept Christianity, neither would they understand democracy. Why then did he continue his merciless war with ever more terrible weapons? This I cannot understand. Truman and MacArthur frequently spoke of God. Why this gap and contradiction between their words and their continual plans to escalate weaponry?

From the time of the founding of Japan until only a century ago, with the importation of a heterogeneous civilization, the population enjoyed a glorious and peaceful history. They were a kind and gentle people with an honest and brave spirit who yet had been invincible to outside attack. Why then does the West not dig deeply into the causes of the unprecedented defeat of Japan? Such research would certainly show something very useful regarding the fate of one civilization. It would provide Westerners with a chance to discover the wonderful unique principle of the philosophy of the Far East. This is the principle that attracted Romain Rolland, the Goncourts,[13] Anatole France, Emerson, Charles Peguy,[14] Pierre Louys,[15] and Lafcadio Hearn.[16] All of these people held a great nostalgia for the vision of a total life concept. Professor Northrop,[17] author of *The Meeting of East and West*, insists that the key for the founding of a world government was already established thousands of years ago and still exists, a treasure waiting to be uncovered, in the mentality of the Far East. He is aware that this consciousness is based on the firm world concept of the unique principle.

Why was MacArthur, who so much loved reading Epictetus, unable to discover this great worldview? Was it perhaps that he also suffered from the weakness of memory that is so common among Westerners?

Beneath all the apparent difficulties in Japan, a country so miserably torn and thrown into chaos after the war, lies nothing but this wonderful and infinite principle. This unique principle, this practical dialectic, is a special treasure that the winner may carry away like a trophy. If the victor is unable to comprehend it, however, the winner will be assimilated by the vanquished just as the Greeks did to their conquerors. This is the dialectical order of the universal constitution. The final and eternal victory goes to the one who has intuitively grasped and become united with the unique principle of universal order.

Chapter 5

Jigaro Kano,
Founder of Kodokan Judo

Jigoro Kano was born in 1860, on the 28th of October, at Mikage—near Kobe—into a very traditional but not very wealthy family. As a child, he was smaller than average and of a frail constitution. He was the third son. In 1881, he graduated from Tokyo University, and in 1882, he founded the Kodokan School of Judo. While still a student, he had researched techniques of resisting defeat by a larger and stronger person. He was born in the midst of a time when there was trouble and confusion at all levels of society. It was the first time in history that Japan had experienced such disorder and, in this way, somewhat resembled France in the eighteenth century.

Kano was born only eight months after the assassination of Tairo Ii outside of Sakuradamon.[18] The Tokugawa prime minister had opened the doors of Japan, which had been closed for three hundred years, and had condemned all the young idealistic leaders who were opposed to his government. Kano was seven years old when the Meiji Restoration was accomplished under the pressure of foreign powers: England, France, Russia, and the United States. In 1871, when he was ten years old, all the *daimyo* (lords) and their territories were overthrown. The samurai, including the masters of *jujitsu*, lost their means of livelihood and had to seek new professions. Many samurai committed suicide. In Tokyo, more than one hundred schools of *jujitsu* were closed.

Kano experienced all these changes and was deeply affected by

51

them. He wished very much to save *jujitsu* and to continue to train himself and polish his ability. He searched out the remaining schools and, one by one, mastered their individual styles. Finally, he founded the first unified school of judo in 1882 with a single student, Tomita, a boy of seventeen years who later reached the highest level, tenth *dan*.

In the beginning, there were no students serious enough about judo to pay monthly dues, and so Kano had to pay the entire expense of the *dojo* himself. He paid everything out of his wages as a professor at Tokyo University and his fees from private lessons. Tomita, for many years, had to wash all the uniforms himself. This was still insufficient. Kano had to earn even more money by translating books and documents for the ministry of education. The economic demands and responsibilities of a new *dojo* were by no means easily met.

Fortunately, however, Japan defeated China, and, in 1897, Lafcadio Hearn published a book in Boston that introduced judo to the West for the first time. These two factors combined to spread the name of judo around the world. In 1901, several important English visitors and about sixty members of the British navy visited the Kodokan. In 1902, Kano sent Yamashita, one of his youngest students, to the United States, and he was of great assistance to President Theodore Roosevelt. In the Russo-Japanese war also, those who had learned judo well played a very important role. With the financial assistance of the wealthy Jewish merchant Jacob Schiff, Japan was able to win the war. From that time on, the reputation of judo continually increased.

Jigoro Kano, the founder of Kodokan, walked one straight path without ever faltering until his death on the Pacific Ocean on May 4, 1938. He was returning from the Olympics in Cairo by way of the United States and was 77 years old at the time. It is rare that such a pioneer lives not only a long but also a happy life.

The basis of his school was: "The Principle of the Best Use of Physical and Spiritual Energy."[19]

His five points for the ideal individual were as follows:

- A person of good health
- A person of justice
- A person who is useful to society
- A person of strong will and courage
- A diligent, hardworking person

The one point he most emphasized was mental and spiritual cultivation. He considered judo as the means to accomplish this. Herein lies the greatest difference between judo and sports, gymnastics, and other kinds of physical exercise.

All of the sciences, as well as all of the Western-style schools, continue to become more and more departmentalized. Each school or department deals only with its own speciality. In the end, they not only cause their own destruction from the inside out, but they also throw humanity into a total state of chaos. The present situation of today's world is the inevitable and unavoidable result of this. In contrast to this, all of the schools of the East are founded upon the *do*, the very same unique and unifying principle that underlies all science, philosophy, religion, and the strategy of peace.

Accordingly, the history of the East is just the opposite of that of the West. It is a history of peace. Japan was at peace from its founding until the twelfth century. During the Nara Period (710-793) and the Heian Period (794-1156), Japanese culture flourished tremendously; various kinds of fine arts were appreciated including poetry, literature, and the tea ceremony. There had not been a single war in Japan from 1600 until the importation of Western civilization (1894).

From the time Japanese people began to import Western civilization and become familiar with Western tools and weapons, they began to believe that they could become even more powerful. Their descent began almost immediately. Prior to that time, they believed it was best to use only judo or the arts of archery and the sword. The way of old Japan, which would never have accepted the premise of rule by power or majority, was overridden by modern education. The Imperial Family always reigned over this docile and all-embracing race. The Japanese race created one great family, and the samurai were the guardians of the royal family that presided over them. After winning the wars with both China and Russia, certain generals, admirals, and soldiers were able to push their way into positions of authority. Herein lies the real ultimate cause of the unprecedented, unconditional surrender of Japan in 1945. Unreasonable force is always toppled in the end; it destroys itself. A society based on force is ephemeral.

Principles of Judo

The essential principle of judo is derived from Chinese military strategy: "The flexible conquer the strong and hard through the use of suppleness." This phrase recalls to us the four following lines of the celebrated philosophy of military strategy.

- The one who is flexible on the outside and firm on the inside will continuously prosper.
- The one who is strong on the outside and weak on the inside will prosper initially but eventually diminish.
- The one who is flexible on the outside and weak on the inside will lose whatever one has inevitably.
- The one who is hard on the outside and strong on the inside will be destroyed sooner or later.

Recall the four combinations, two yang and two yin elements. The two yang are firmness (hardness) and strength. The two yin are flexibility and weakness. Sun Tsu, the most famous philosopher of military strategy in China, devotes the first chapter of his strategic classic, *The Art of War*,[20] to the establishment of peace through the *tao*. He goes on to explain further the nature of the *tao*: "The *tao* is that which teaches all people and nations how to rise above all difficulties and fears. It is the actual method of philosophy that guarantees total freedom."

And yet, how is one to actually realize these combinations of yin and yang, suppleness and power, both physiologically and psychologically? What educational method can accomplish this? How are yin (a flexible and peaceful personality) and yang (a strong and unshakable will) to be harmonized within our physical body?

In the *I Ching* (ancient Chinese classic of divination) it states, "Pure water possesses the gentleness of a mother's caress and extends life-giving benevolence to all things of both the animal and the vegetable kingdoms. Nevertheless, it has the undefeatable power to erode the earth's surface and even rocks, without fighting at all." By what method can we possibly train human beings to gain power resembling that of the nature of water? What kind of hammering is necessary for human beings to learn how to change their constitution at will? Everyone wishes that they could change their constitution and become perfect and matchless. If this were possible we would be able to alter our destiny as well. We must, first of all, grasp the connection between our physiological constitution and our spiritual nature or quality. It is of these things that no one speaks, not Sun Tsu, not Lao Tsu, not the Buddha, not Jesus Christ. Kano, as well, mentions nothing about it. This is the common deficiency of all great people. Although their teachings are based on beautiful ideals, they have not really solved the problem of how to effectively and practically realize these ideals. Everyone knows that it is both necessary and desirable to establish a mental and physical constitution that is externally supple and internally resistant and strong. Furthermore, everyone recognizes the need for mutual love, brotherhood, altruism, loyalty, and goodwill. The problem remains, however, as to the method or methods through which this can be accomplished or turned into a practical reality. All of the various schools give years of education in these precepts. Then, after graduating from school, each person must discover how to practically realize these goals. Quite often those who have been well educated commit far greater blunders than those who haven't been to school at all.

There is no animal that would attempt to imitate the foolish behavior of humans. Among the animal kingdom, it is the human alone who is unable to practically realize these necessary conditions of life. All other animals master them intuitively. When other animals must fight, they don't manufacture firearms or atomic bombs. Although they sometimes fight among themselves, they never seek an aggressive encounter with human beings. If such an encounter should occur, the blame inevitably lies with the human.

If you should be stung by an innocent bee, which seeks only after a sweet and sugary smell, it is your own fault. The composition of your blood and consequently of your entire constitution is saturated with excess sweetness and the sugary taste. Is not the laxity of your personality and the weakness of your physiological makeup dependent on the quality and composition of your blood and entire constitution? If you find the sting of a bee intolerable, perhaps you should understand this as a divine warning. This is a signal that your life is in danger. If you visit Africa and are attacked by crocodiles, it is you who have invaded their natural habitat without reserve or warning and thereby caused them to become afraid and angry.

If, for example, your lungs are overrun with tiny microscopic microbes and bacteria, this is proof that your constitution is weak and has very little resistance. This is your own fault also. You have certain responsibilities. It is you who are the criminal. You continued, over a long period of time, to follow the wrong kind of diet. You must correct this error. If you seek to do so by taking medicines or depending on the assistance of others, you will only compound the crimes you have already committed against nature. Jesus Christ never depended on any medicines, even those natural medicines of the Far East.

In this universe, from the largest stars and planets to the microscopic basic elements, all things conform to cyclical spiralic form. In actual fact, this form is established by the interaction of two circular energies that are antagonistic to each other. To our limited senses, whether these be large stars or tiny electrons, this whirling movement appears to be undulating orbits of diffraction of electrons or the elliptical orbiting of fixed stars. In actual fact, however, all of these bodies are moving in logarithmic spirals.

Each of these spirals has the same qualities at their center. These qualities are heat, centripetality, hardness, and resistance. In opposition to this, the periphery has the opposite characteristics of cold, centrifugality, softness, little resistance, and fragility.

Observed from the view of electromagnetic energy, the center and the periphery are the opposite extremes of yin and yang. The above is an initial attempt to create a cosmological explanation of the universe, but it will be verified one day by ultramodern science.

It is extremely interesting to note that within the philosophy of Sun Tsu, as well as the principles of all respectable schools of the *do*, this cosmological and electronic explanation of universal construction is clearly indicated. Within the *do* is the origin of astrology and of all the dialectical theories of Democritus, Hippocrates, the *I Ching*, Lao Tsu, and Jesus. Unfortunately, however, over the centuries all of this original theory has been misinterpreted time and time again until the remaining teaching bears little resemblance to the original. In its degenerated form, this original wisdom becomes little more than another form of superstition or regresses still further to become the mystical doctrine of various ideological groups with some small semblance of supernatural ability. Modern science itself is, in fact, no more than a nostalgia for magic.

The Way of Medicine

Far Eastern medicine, *ido*, is an approach to physical and mental health through correct and nourishing food. It utilizes no method except diet and has nothing to do with bloody operations. Moxibustion, acupuncture, and palm healing are only symptomatic treatments. True therapy is dietetic.

Even so, this does not mean Western medicine is an adversary. This would be impossible because the purpose of Far Eastern medicine is to establish the physiological foundation for social, political, and economic freedom. Wouldn't it truly be a wonderful thing if humankind would have no more need of medicine at all? Far Eastern medicine is not only curative; it is also for the education of society. It is not merely a method of treatment. The *do* of medicine eliminates the need for suffering from sickness. The *do* of medicine teaches all people how they can live in health, freedom, and happiness. It teaches us practical theory that can be easily applied to our daily lives. It gives us intuitive wisdom for life and a view of universal order through which we can logically deduce life's reality. It never makes use of complex, expensive, and cruel implements to accomplish its purpose. Far Eastern medicine is a gentle and living wisdom for all people. It is a permanent individual revolution that takes place through everyday biological and physiological education leading to a lively and enjoyable life for each and every person.

Far Eastern medicine is, in its nature, close to Hygeia, goddess of health in Greek mythology. It takes care of education, economy, philosophy, and government. To understand why this is so, one has only to look at the name by which the great doctors in Japan, China, and Korea are referred to, that is, *kokushi*, "the hand that physiologically leads the people in a free and happy country."

"To control a larger and stronger person through the use of suppleness and flexibility" is the principle of Kano's judo. It has nothing to do with killing or annihilating one's enemies. It means to attract and lead one's adversaries and all of those affiliated with them into a world of peace and harmony. Once having entered such a world, there is no longer any need for self-defense or the taking up of weapons for the purpose of mutual destruction.

Judo is, above all, a cooperative activity where those opposed to each other are united by the common goal of polishing themselves as well as bringing each other to perfection through actual training. They strive to realize peace and freedom through actual training. It is the spirit of Abraham Lincoln at Gettysburg. Neither peace nor freedom can be established by the elimination of the other side. Exclusivity, egoism, and monopoly are now and always have been empty of any value. They are utterly meaningless and useless. It is almost like killing oneself by mistake. Within this all-embracing universe, even the smallest amount of exclusivity is a great crime.

There are sufficient examples throughout history. There is not even one example of an empire established by the enslavement or annihilation of the adversary that has lasted even one century in peace. Medicine is the same. The medicine that merely fortifies symptomatic treatments, attempting to eliminate bacteria or virus, which are as illusory as astral spirits, never seeks to cure our real faults or insufficiencies. This medicine can never discover the real cause of sickness.

Nonchalantly and with spiritual color blindness, we continue to invent more and more devilish medicines such as the treatments of Ehrlich, Flemming, Banting, and Best;[21] the vaccines of Jenner and Pasteur; and streptomycin, penicillin, and the sulfa drugs. According to Epictetus, Jesus, Buddha, Gandhi, and Hygeia, unhappiness is entirely our own responsibility. Despite the fact that those who are unhappy or lacking in moral qualities can be easily persuaded into changing themselves, people continue instead to produce weapons of war with which to annihilate their enemies.

This is just like the competitive marathon that goes on without solution between medicine and sickness. Sickness is always in the lead. Microbes develop and new incurable diseases continue to be created from the so-called cure for the old ones. Among these are the various cancers as well as mental and moral illnesses. War is only one more symptom of these self-inflicted illnesses, and its escalation already threatens the entire human race. Far Eastern medicine is a completely different kind of therapy. Judo is one example of how to transform the most powerful enemy (which is also the least powerful), without killing or subjugation or the use of any weapon, into a good friend.

If judo can accomplish such a feat, why then is it not possible for us, without creating the dangerous repercussions from using various technical and scientifically complicated methods, to make friends with the smallest and most minute of enemies, the microbes and viruses and all of the basic elements that constitute the ultimate cause of illness?

To study judo is to gain possession of the most practical and yet ultimate medicine for curing all sickness. It is to study and eventually grasp the most effective and useful principle of principles, the order of the universe. Standing at the entrance doorway of judo and the way of medicine, humanity is on the threshold of the heaven known as peace and freedom.

But did Kano also practice the way of medicine? There is no way to be absolutely certain of this. Nevertheless, the fact that he was loved by everyone and lived a very happy natural life span of nearly eighty years definitely indicates that this was the case. He was a man who lived his life from beginning to end without modification or straying from his original intention, and he also had the rare quality of being willing to relive it with the greatest of joy. If one would be unwilling to joyfully relive his or her life exactly as it was, without changing anything, it means one has lived the life of an unhappy slave or a criminal.

Throughout his life, Kano was never detested or even disliked. On the contrary, he was loved by all even after his death. He realized all his dreams freely, pursuing whatever he liked and to whatever degree he chose. This means that he understood the principle of principles, the order of the universe, the constitution of universal law or *michi*, *do*, the way of life. Kano, just as all sages and great masters, had made the principles of a happy life an integral part of his being. There is no one who can live this kind of completely happy life and be forever loved by everyone without such knowledge and understanding.

Dialectical Opposites

George Bernard Shaw said, "He who knows cannot teach and he who teaches does not know." People who spend the majority of their time teaching will find it difficult to divide their time conveniently for learning. The study of theory is a yin endeavor, whereas teaching others is yang. These two are exactly opposite. The person who can learn and teach without one obstructing the other is a rare individual indeed. Opposites in equal proportions neutralize each other. To begin with, everyone's constitution contains a totally different balance of yin and yang. Everyone always has either yin or yang in excess.

It goes without saying that the character of learning and understanding, rather than teaching, would be predominant if one wishes to continually increase one's joy and satisfaction in life. Nevertheless, according to the order of the universe, the human biological constitution is yang at the center and yin at the surface. This is one example indicating the great logarithmical spiral of the universe; within this spiral, all things are born, exist, grow, change, and disappear and reappear. If, according to your daily food, both of these circumstances are continually nourished and strengthened, you should be able to develop both sides to your maximum potential. Let us, therefore, make some slight revision and improvement in the aforementioned statement by Bernard Shaw: "The one who knows can also teach and the one who teaches can also know if one has the compass." The compass is the principle of life, universal order, or an intuitive universal view of the order of nature, society, and humanity.

Nothing is easier than this. Imagine the body as the center of our environment and the universe as the periphery of our body. These two are one inseparable reality. The greater your field of activity (centrifugality or exterior environment), the stronger your center (centripetality or internal environment) becomes. The person with the greatest radial scope of activity, infinite yin power, also has the greatest yang power and vice versa. This is the very person who has realized both freedom and happiness. This is a person who has yang on the inside and yin on the outside.

Kano, thanks to his mother, who observed the precepts of nature's order, was blessed with just such a constitution. That is to say, he was the most avaricious and egotistical person! If you have the greatest yang (greed, egoism, forcefulness), you also have the potential to someday gain the greatest yin (compassion, philanthropy, and love). The most evil person may even become one of the highest virtue, while a weak friend may do you no good at all. If you are able to change your enemy into a friend, it is because you are making use of the dialectical compass of which we are speaking. That person will become your most necessary and valued friend.

The thing that people tend to neglect the most is the most important of all things—that is, the harmonious unification of these two environments, the inner and the outer. We tend to think of the surface of our body as our periphery or limited boundary, but this is nothing more than a selfish pre-Copernican illusion. Boundaries do not exist between countries, individuals, or the individual and his environment. There are no boundaries between the wind, the rain, the sun, oxygen, energy, time, space, and all the essential elements of our constitution.

The concept of boundaries is the idea of monopoly or the exclusive possession of property. This is a kind of spiritual and moral color blindness or nearsightedness. Because of it, the world is full of hostile phantoms. This kind of thinking is a physiological product born from a paralyzed and decaying instinct. This monopolistic thinking is, however, more of a physiological variation than an actual illness. It is not yet sufficient cause for distress. It is merely the activity of a weak and underdeveloped center (centripetality). This center must be able to attract the periphery (centrifugality) even as the periphery is increasingly expanding. All things are brought to a final conclusion by the dialectical construction of the universe.

The most important point, in any case, is to assimilate the two poles—North and South, East and West, center and periphery, the two contending sides of a single whole—into one body. Our enemies are the very reason for our happiness. Without them, our happiness would cease to exist. Happiness is when you succeed in converting an adversary into a valued and eternal friend. Your emotional joy is uncontrollable, and you smile from the inside; you are filled with vitality, and yet your feeling is delicate and gentle. Such was the happiness of Kano. The most lamentable thing is that his creation, the Kodokan, which literally means "the place where one studies the absolute, infinite, and unique principle of the order of the universe and the philosophy of the *tao*," is no longer discussed or studied. It has become nothing more than a mere sports center, as that is the emphasis that has been placed on the practice of judo. Perhaps this can be called dialectical fate.

Chapter 6

Morihei Ueshiba, Founder of Aikido

Morihei Ueshiba was born December 14,1880 in the small village of Tanabe on the coast of Wakayama prefecture. It is a warm (yang) province most concerned with the fishing industry and raising Japanese tangerines (*mikan*). He was the only son among one younger and two older sisters. He was the third child of the four children. His father, Yoroku, had long been the head of the county union and was highly respected by those living in the surrounding area as well as in his own village.

The young Ueshiba left his village at fifteen years of age and went to Tokyo where he studied various schools of the *do*. He was small of stature (5 feet tall, 132 pounds) but had robust health and quite formidable strength. Even at seventy-one, he was still strong and youthful. His student, Minoru Mochizuki, slightly before his 1951 voyage to Europe aboard the *Marseillaise* at the age of 44, one day suddenly, with full force, attacked the aging master who was at that time sitting formally on his knees. Mochizuki was unable, however, to make the master fall. When Ueshiba was sixty-one, the *Asahi News Journal* made a film of him practicing aikido. He was surrounded by fifteen judo practitioners of fifth degree or higher. When they all attempted to pin him down, he threw them all with a single miraculous movement.

Such ability can hardly be called less than miraculous. All who visited his *dojo* could see such techniques and their endless variations. This is a common trait that can be found among all the great masters of the *do*. It is the same with the masters of yoga, whose art is often thought to be the likeness of magic. Professor Eugen Herrigel, as was previously described, witnessed a similar miraculous event at the *dojo* of Master Awa and later recorded it in detail in his book on Japanese archery.

Ueshiba is a self-taught man, a person of strongly independent and autonomous character. He studied neither Western sciences nor philosophy, yet he speaks in quite intellectual terms and his students are frequently at a loss to solve the meaning behind his words. He is also a poet. His teaching is not of a verbal nature but one based primarily on action and the transmission of direct experience. And as in all other schools of the *do*, speaking during training or speaking out of turn is forbidden. Silence dominates everything. It is, in this sense, a bit like a monastery. In the *Manyoshu,* it was stated by the great poet Hitomaro, "Yamato [the ancient name of Japan] is a country where the value of the spoken word is not acknowledged."

I am here to decry, however, this taboo against speaking, and yet I am obliged to be, and soon will have to become, silent. Why is this? The more people speak, the farther they separate themselves from the *do*, the age-old and time-honored path that has evolved silently since before the dawn of history. This silence or space is recognized in the various schools of traditional Japanese painting, exactly opposite from Western painting in every way. These great paintings utilize the fewest brush strokes possible. One such painter is Sesshu, who died in 1506 at the age of eighty-seven. Utamaro and Hiroshige (the latter died in 1849 at the age of ninety) are rather more modem. It seems that the Goncourts were unaware of the earlier schools of classic painting that expressed the *do*.

At this writing, Ueshiba lives in his small and humble house on a hill in the countryside of Ibaraki prefecture. In the space adjoining the *dojo*, two or three of his student-disciples are living together and training with the master. He is also a great farmer, cultivating his fields alone in the traditional Japanese fashion, without any machines. Last year, he harvested some 1,400 pounds of rice; 17,500 pounds of potatoes; several hundred pounds of *azuki* beans; buckwheat, wheat, and vegetables. There was no one in his area who could match his efforts.

According to my diagnosis when I met him, his heart was slightly weak, but even so, compared to my own students at Maison Ignoramus,[22] he was much stronger and had no health problems at all.

Where does his physical, physiological, and spiritual strength and sturdiness come from? His will is like iron. He is seemingly uneducated and appears to be a pleasant, amicable, aging farmer.

Let me introduce a certain episode to you. In 1930, when Mochizuki opened his *dojo* at Shizuoka, he invited Master Ueshiba to attend the opening. He attended accompanied by ten of his higher-ranking students. After the ceremony, the younger fifth and sixth *dan* students, full of youthful energy, accompanied the master to show him the beautiful sights of the countryside. They climbed up the Nippon Daira plateau (an ascent of five miles) along a path across the tea fields. The master, in traditional *hakama* (ceremonial dress) and *geta* (wooden clogs), climbed the hills almost as if running and the students, unable to follow, were left behind. They attempted to make a shortcut through the tea fields. Seeing this, the tea farmers began yelling and taking up bamboo staffs to drive them out of the fields. The young students found this amusing and half in jest began to prepare themselves for a fight. The farmers continued to descend upon them from the summit. At that moment, both opposing sides were taken aback by the sudden appearance of Master Ueshiba. Seeing the problem, he had hastily retraced his steps from some five hundred yards ahead and placed himself between the two groups. Facing towards the farmers, he crouched down on his hands and knees and bowed formally to them.

"Everyone, please accept my humble and formal apology. There is no acceptable excuse for what we have done. As you can see before you, I am at your disposal. These fellows are my young students, and they confused the path because I climbed up it too quickly."

The young farmers, simple and honest, were dumbfounded to see an old man resembling the prime minister bowing down on the ground before them, and they began to apologize for their own hasty behavior and short temper.

The students were prepared for a severe reprimanding when they reached the summit, but the master spoke to them instead in a jovial manner: "The work of a farmer is difficult and tiring, and yet they make very little money. Their job is never finished, and their wages are never enough. In comparison to this, the master as well as the students of the do work very little and are generally lazy. It is hardly just, is it? Ha, ha, ha, ha..."

The iron will, healthy body, and soft, flexible personality of Ueshiba are truly enigmatic. It is probably due to his strong constitution that he is able to realize his ambitions, and this is also the basis of his personality. He has never made any propaganda for his own teachings. He always avoids being conspicuous. He even confessed to me one day that he had a desire to hide himself in the distant mountains, away from people, in order to perfect himself.

He owes the formulation of his constitution to the following factors:

- Yang geographical and climatic conditions. His birthplace was exposed to salty sea winds and hot sunshine. There was little humidity and a shortage of drinking water. The terrain being rocky, it supported few vegetables and relatively few fruits in spite of the warm climate.
- His yang embryological period (March to December). In other words, out of the nine months of pregnancy, six months (mid-March to mid-September) were warm (yang) months and the remaining time (October to December) were cold (yin) months. Furthermore, during the yin months, his mother was busy with harvesting activities. Therefore, during the time he developed in his mother's womb, he received much yang power. Born in the cold month of December, both mother and child had to take in less liquid (yin) to protect themselves from the cold weather. Also during winter time, she had to eat root vegetables. Thus, his mother's milk was low in liquid content, which also made him more yang.

- Since childhood, his body was trained by hard work.
- For the first fifteen years of his life with his family, he lived a life of difficulty and sometimes neediness (*vivere parvo*[23]). In Tokyo, after leaving his family at fifteen to study judo and other martial arts, he had to endure a very meager existence bordering on poverty.
- His life of hard labor in the extremely bitter cold of the wilderness of Hokkaido (1912-1921).

His mother, like all the farming women of Japan's rural villages, was a very hardworking woman. His father was the same. Morihei himself was, as a result, also a hardworking person. Salt causes the muscles to contract, making one's constitution yang, and salt was abundant in his environment—in the air and the vegetables and grains. Moreover, he worked hard physically and didn't drink much of any liquid. The combination of these factors made his constitution all the more yang. The hard work, which he endured from childhood, the yang quality of the local food and water, no availability of meat or sweets and few fruits—these things make up the essence of *vivere parvo*, the secret for the formation of a strong innerly yang constitution with good quality yin on the surface.

To work very hard with a minimal standard of living is the very way to consolidate a firm constitution based on a mild and peaceful personality.

Judo is not a sport; nevertheless, it can be practiced as one. Aikido, on the other hand, can in no way be utilized as a sport. Ueshiba hated making it into a spectacle or using it for public display. Aikido cannot be classified as a method or theory of martial technique, and it cannot be classified together with gymnastics or other such games. It is a practical aesthetic. Furthermore, it is impossible to learn aikido in large groups. It can only be passed down directly from a master or senior student. If this is not the case, there can be great risk of broken bones and other serious injuries. Senior students of similar rank can practice together. This, however, is for the purpose of polishing and perfecting their technique as well as making it free-flowing, harmonious, and beautiful. It is forbidden for beginners to practice together.

Had Lafcadio Hearn been able to witness the training of Ueshiba sensei's students, he would have been astonished. The practice of aikido is aesthetic and beautiful to watch. It leaves one with a pleasant and agreeable feeling. In judo, by comparison, one tends to see only fierce confrontation.

Ueshiba sensei forbade competition for the sake of determining superiority. The goal of aikido is to become aware of your own insufficiencies, of the transitoriness and ephemerality of human victory, of human weakness, and the insignificant foolishness of vanity. It is a philosophical and cosmological education for the purpose of becoming happy and free. It is by no means a mere competitive sport for testing the superiority of power, muscles, or animal dexterity. Rather it is spiritual, philosophical, moral, and cosmological. It is a methodical treatise on peace. It avoids all the cruel, barbaric, and futile conflicts that always lead only to more of the same. It is the avoidance of massacre. It is a means of self-defense that relies exclusively on the art of receiving, never on the art of attack.

Aikido pacifies violent attacks, immobilizing the enemy by the least and simplest physical technique. It utilizes exactly the same principle as the school of flower arrangement (*kado*), where one arranges flowers according to the nature of the flowers themselves, without employing any artificial techniques and using the scissors as little as possible. *Kado* is an art like medicine or the art of longevity, enabling the cut flowers to live even as much as five or six times longer than flowers in the natural environment. Even the chrysanthemum, which usually dries up quickly under normal temperatures, can be preserved for up to a month through the techniques of *kado*. There is even a special technique for cutting flowers without injuring them.

It was written by Yutang that primitive Orientals have a great deal of difficulty comprehending the reasons why people engage in competitive sports activities. What is to be gained or accomplished by their practice? If they are solely for the purpose of developing muscular strength, they are strictly for pleasure, nothing more, and altogether useless. Case by case, according to individual constitutions, they may actually be quite detrimental.

Let me introduce here one more episode: The famous boxer Horiguchi, nicknamed "The Piston," came one day to the Ueshiba *dojo* requesting a match of the two different arts. The master invited him to attack with his full force and power. The boxer attacked violently, continuously throwing the straight and crushing blows for which he was known, to the chest of the master. The master then reached out and struck both of Horiguchi's arms from the outside. It was a supple and yet sharp blow that was so fast no one really saw it. The boxer had no time even to be amazed. He fell to the ground, both of his arms broken Horiguchi had to be cared for in a hospital for a period of two months.

It is Ueshiba's intention to completely eliminate the competition that also lends itself to exhibitionism. This is because aikido is the firm and eternal foundation on which peace and harmony rest. It is a philosophy based on a universal concept; in the largest meaning of the word, it is a religion.

Thus, aikido is much more than a technique for strengthening the body. It constantly employs the use of the dialectical principle of yin and yang and, through actual practice, aims at perfecting one's character through a universal conception or cosmology. Yin and yang are the unique tools of this magnificent universe. They are, together in their unified and dynamic reality, the compass that makes possible the realization of a free and peaceful humanity.

Chapter 7

The Order of the Universe

Complementary antagonism is the definitive characteristic of this illusory and relative world. The relative world exists as an infinitesimal geometric point of incessant change within the one absolute and infinite world, beyond time-space and without limitation or restriction. This relative world is a theatre of performances in which all the tiny and ephemeral parts are woven together in endless variations. The great universe itself, however, is one unified existence without beginning or end. The latter is an ocean of absolute infinite expansion, while the former is a world of fleeting and transitory sense data that is continually multiplying. The universe is infinite not only in time and expansive space, but also within the geometrical constitution of each of the individual elements or parts existing within that great expanse.

The drama of this relative world, however, is not without order. It is not mere chaos. There is a clear lineage of natural order that each and every person, primitive or modem, is living within and according to. For example: summer and winter; heat and cold; day and night; humidity and dryness; male and female; beginning and end; activity and passivity; ascending and descending; growth and diminution; blossoming and withering; centripetal and centrifugal force; constriction and dilation; construction and destruction; rest and movement; fast and slow—all of these opposing factors are in constant contrast and conflict. Taken together, these opposites are but the two ends of a spectrum. Although opposing each other, they are also attracted to each other under the influence of a superior force;

they keep crossing and exchanging their positions. These opposites are, in fact, the very reason why so-called evolution goes on within nature at an increasing rate of speed.

When these opposing factors are lined up in the above manner, it is as Shakespeare recognized in his *Troilus and Cressida*: "The heavens themselves, the planets and our central globe follow conditions of degree, priority, rank, regularity of the course, proportion, season, shape, role, and custom in an invariable order."

What a great man, this Shakespeare! What is it that really constitutes greatness? It is an awareness of the thread of order that runs through and unifies all the various manifestations and changes, both visible and invisible, on this earth and throughout the universe, including the data collected by our senses ranging from love to war. The French have a well-developed awareness of the order of the universe. This is shown in their language, which divides all nouns into male and female gender.

A great person is happy. Heaven belongs to him or to her. One who is great and strong does not engage in verbal disputes. One doesn't attack or ridicule. One embraces everything. One doesn't view hardship as suffering, but rather rises above it and uses it for personal growth and improvement. A truly great person is one who, with his or her own intuitive judgment of universal order, unites all the various miracles of life and nature. This is like the tailor dedicated to the making of an elegant suit, assembling all the material and binding it together by concentrated effort. People such as this are pure and seem to be invisible, blending through everything. Their heart and mind are the reality of peace, and their total activity is justice and freedom.

Those who are antagonistic and constantly in conflict with each other are only one end of a bar magnet. They are antagonistic but, at the same time, parts of the same magnet. They are also attracted to each other and exchange their magnetic flow. In reality, the activity of one side is just the same as that of the other. In any case, even though it may be undetectable to most people, all things are united by the single, thin thread of order that eternally controls the universe. Many thousands of years ago in China, this thread of order was given the name of tao, which, translated into more modern terms, is divine knowledge or cosmic consciousness. I have reissued this wisdom for the twentieth century, calling it "the order of the universe" or "the order of the universal constitution." This is necessary because the symbolic language of the primitive mind no longer penetrates our consciousness in these modern times. Some of the words in these ancient languages indicate gender through yin and yang.

The Order of the Universe in Seven Logical Principles

So that all people can understand the order that exists behind the seeming chaos of this world, I would like to present you with seven extremely fundamental and universal laws. If any of these are unacceptable to you, I would appreciate your criticism. It is quite possible that my manner of expression may make it difficult for you to understand my meaning clearly.

1. Whatever has a beginning has an end (antagonism in time: the principle of inversion). That which has a beginning is inevitably proceeding toward its opposite. Beginning and end are always opposed to each other: birth-death; formation-transformation; poverty-wealth; meeting-separation; having-losing, etc.

In this way, all of these various functions are inverted forms of their opposite. All things in this relative world, at a greater or lesser pace, will eventually conform to this law.

If there is anything that does not conform to this law, it belongs to the absolute, infinite world. Such a thing, however, is exceedingly rare. You must be extremely careful in order to detect the invisible and infinite thread that runs through and connects all things.

2. That which has a front has a back (antagonism in matter: the principle of *omote-ura*, front and back in Japanese). Front and back are opposites, and they are also complementary. There is nothing in this world that has one without the other. The surface of a Gobelin tapestry and its reverse side are inseparable and yet opposed A new weapon invites another superior weapon; profit is always accompanied by some aspect of loss. The streets of modern cities are filled

with crime. Joy and suffering are twins.

3. No two things are identical (principle of difference). There are no two identical things in this world. Mountains, rivers, rocks, states and countries, the earth and other planets, the sun and stars, people: all are unique.

4. The larger and greater the front, the larger and greater the back (the principle of balance).

When one reaps great profits in some way, one inevitably receives great losses in another. Great progress is accompanied by great degeneration. One example is the striking contrast of modem civilization and nuclear warfare. The legal system and the police are always running a competitive marathon with crime. It is the same with Western medicine and disease.

5. Change (differentiation or movement) as well as stability (state of temporary equilibrium as two opposing forces exchange their energy and direction) are products of the two fundamental, universal, and dialectic forces of yin (centrifugality) and yang (centripetality) confronting each other (principle of dual origin).

The forces of yin and yang are interpreted as cold-hot; dark-light; acid-alkaline; dilation-constriction; ascent-descent; negative-positive; feminine-masculine, respectively. These are all antagonistic and at the same time complementary.

Everything is in a state of constant, incessant change. All is fluctuating, volatile, and ephemeral. All is engaged and in motion. Motion, differentiation, joining together, and decomposition are all nothing more than the various processes of change through which all things must inevitably pass. Mountains are waves that rise and fall within empty space and then subside and vanish into nothing. Change is everything. Balance, equilibrium, or harmonization are the point where two different directions meet and exchange their respective energies. All changes, as well as so-called balance or equilibrium, are produced and given life by the intersecting of opposites. The resulting scene is then projected onto the screen of the absolute or infinity.

6. These opposing factors are the right and left hands of the one,

absolute, eternal infinity (principle of polarization).

Because yin and yang are in reality complementary, all phenomena have a dialectical constitution made of these two opposing factors. All physical phenomena contain a central point that gathers all peripheral elements toward its center. Furthermore, all chemical elements are made up of two groups that continually contend with each other. For this reason, one uses the reactionary changes of opposing factors such as acid and alkaline and heat and cold alternatively for physical or chemical analysis and synthesis. Without antagonism, there is also nothing complementary. Yin and yang are the two hands that create, sustain, and destroy in order to produce anew everything that exists in the world. Therefore, all things existing are inevitably relative, antagonistic, and, at the same time, complementary. Where there is no conflict, there is also no harmony. Where there is no contradiction, there is also no agreement. Therefore, every thesis is progressing towards antithesis in order to synthesize and create a new thesis.

I believe, at this point, it should be obvious that the above six principles, all of the relative world, completely destroy all the old laws or theories. These are, after all, of no use whatsoever in solving the disputes and quarrels of everyday and family life, much less international conflicts, which require an even larger perspective in order to understand. Formal logic is an extremely sensory and simple-minded Western invention. It is one of the most ignorant examples of thought to come out of Kant's style. The law of identity is demolished without a sound by the principle of inversion, as is the law of the mean by the principle of balance.

7. The principle of polarized oneness. The infinite universe, the world of oneness, is constant and unchanging. It is limitless and omniscient and eternal. It gives birth to all things within the limited world of relative existence. It is through the power of the one that all things are nurtured, raised up to their prime, destroyed, and again reborn.

This oneness may be referred to as God, the all-knowing, all-powerful, and ever-present one; the ruler of the universe; that primal force that is uncreated and without beginning or end; the infinite, eternal, one.

Principles one through six appeal to the five senses. They are a sketch of the order of the relative world. They are the most fundamental principles underlying the entire manifest world, from the earth we live on to the great expanse of the universe. In contrast to these, the seventh principle is a sketch of the parental source of yin and yang, the ultimate cause of the universe itself.

These seven principles do not change. Together, they constitute the order of the universe, and this order is the only eternal truth in our world. This is the foundation of all logic or theory. In fact, the only school of logic that is truly universal and eternal is that which is correctly established on this order. All things ideological or social, as well as physical, that are not based on this order will sooner or later be destroyed by their own inertia, fall into the chaos that they have invited, and finally perish altogether.

All scientific and cultural laws are based on the laws of physical nature, which, in turn, are based on the order of the universe. This order is the creator of all the various complex manifestations of this world and, therefore, seems on the surface to be extremely complex, while in actuality it is quite simple. If its essence is not understood, it will be impossible to establish world government or a world constitution. If we intuitively grasp this unique truth, the order of the universe, and make it a part of our own being, we will be able to manifest whatever we dream. "Know the truth and the truth will set you free." "Seek first the kingdom of heaven and its justice and all else shall be added unto you." Matthew 6:33.

The kingdom of heaven of which Jesus spoke is none other than the absolute, eternal, infinite world spoken of in the seventh principle. The justice of this kingdom is none other than the eternally unchanging order of the universe that guides and leads all things to their intended perfection. If you once make this order into your own understanding, you will be able to resolve all conflicts and make all antagonisms complementary. Jesus and Lao Tsu were among those few great sages who discovered the universal order. Jesus called it "divine justice" and stated that "All words are from the mouth of God." The famous words, "Know thyself, the kingdom is within you," mean you must know yourself and the order of the universe, the dialectical constitution of life itself. (How is it that you were created by this order and by what means was the life force itself brought into being?)

Now you should be able to comprehend that the words of Epictetus, "Everyone is happy; if not, it is their own fault," are exactly correct. The fault or error is in not having practically realized this dialectical order of the universe. False and mistaken education is an invention of the evil minority who are in a governing position. The rule of the people is always in the hands of more yin or more yang groups, each in their alternative turns. If a ruler does not wish to succumb to this tendency and be overthrown by antagonistic forces, the government or regime has only to be chosen with a correct proportion of these opposing groups. But then it would be necessary to establish a new Copernican method of electing leaders.

At last, now you have the key to the kingdom of heaven, the order of the universe. But you still do not know how to use it. It is a shame, but I am forced to abbreviate this explanation greatly in this work.

Chapter 7

The Compass of Happiness

There are many precious books that have been written by saints and wise people with the purpose of instructing us in solving the riddle of true freedom, peace, and happiness and how to attain them. There are also endless declarations and sermons on independence, brotherhood, love, and God. Nevertheless, no one in history even up to this present day, in any country whatsoever, has ever seen or lived a totally complete and happy life.

Mahatma Gandhi, whose life was dedicated to nonviolence, died in a violent fashion. I wonder if Woodrow Wilson would be happy if he could catch a glimpse today of the state of all his shattered dreams? Could Hilty, the saint of Switzerland, if he saw those who loved to read his books living in fear of nuclear weapons and war, be altogether happy seeing their miserable state? Would he be able to find a single one of his students in a really happy state? Bergson received great admiration from both students and scholars and yet how many of them will become happy after studying his philosophy? Upton Sinclair delighted his readers with his huge ten volumes of *Lanny Budd* in which he exposed the behind-the-scenes activities on the stage of world government. For this, his poor readers paid him in advance. But what have they gained? They were able to pass a few hours wringing their hands over some interesting and disturbing reading. Is it really much more than this? Was Einstein contented and happy when he saw the world's people trembling in fear? Even if this were the case, could such complacent happiness continue for more than ten or twenty years?

Reading history, one learns that there have been many who were great in their lifetimes, and yet, in our time, they are already forgotten or no longer loved or respected. Some, like Charles and John Wesley, lived very long lives and are also loved by many people today. Buddha, Jesus, and Mohammed are the same. Confucius died a tragic death, but he is loved by certain of his countrymen even today. These founders of various religions lived much happier lives than the above-mentioned greats of science, literature, and politics. Nevertheless, in spite of their self-conversion and their own teachings, there is hardly a one who has really become "as a small child." If there are any among those great saints who could accomplish this, they did so by their own power; they had no need to be led by teachers. Such people were born with a natural inclination towards self-development.

The average person having no inclination towards self-development regardless of the opportunities that may be presented, it is no wonder that there is no end to the unhappiness exemplified by war, sickness, fear, quarreling, hardship, crime, unrest, and the use of brute force to accomplish one's own selfish ends, either in the past or in this present modern-day society. Further, no one knows the principal cause behind all of this misfortune and unhappiness, and no one is capable of a powerful critique or attack on this problem through constructive criticism, above all through self-criticism or self-reflection.

People are lacking the compass that would enable them to judge and choose the best method and course of action concerning every kind of difficulty and contradiction. In the end, the majority of the populace have become run-of-the-mill "Milquetoast"[24] types of people. On the opposite pole stand the leaders of the minority groups. The average person, Mr. or Mrs. Milquetoast, is without direction, and the minority leaders have become the adventurous captains of the ship of life. This passenger ship, however, always sails in uncharted seas, and the captain's past experience, as well as his compass, are of no use. It is, therefore, quite natural and common that a voyage in the rough seas of life ends in shipwreck. The human power of judgment and decision, understanding and criticism, as well as the mind of self-reflection, is lacking a basic standard or principle—a compass or way to make balance. All of these things are inevitably mistaken, therefore, from the beginning to the end.

For thousands of years, the saints, the wise, and the scholars have attempted to unravel and elucidate the principle of one riddle, that of love. How to love and be loved like small children? When one loves or wants to love, there always seems to be a contradiction between that love and the freedom that everybody also wishes to obtain and no one wants to sacrifice. It seems the two cannot be established side by side. Parents' love for their children, a man's love for a woman or vice versa, is not necessarily love. This may, at times, be only one kind of sentimentality or egoism. It is well understood that love is a beautiful thing, and everyone really wishes to love and be loved. And yet, due to the territorial battle between love and freedom, they are in a state of confusion. No one knows how to solve the conflict between love and freedom.

Wise people and scholars of ancient times point out to us very forcibly that the connection between these two things is, in fact, the only exit from the problem. They point this out in different words, but they are all of the same mind. People cannot seem to understand that the principle of liberty and that of love are one and the same. It is ignorance of this principle that causes all the unhappiness and tragedy. Whence comes this ignorance? It is due to: 1) Bad memory, color blindness of the memory; 2) Weakened powers of reason, color blindness of the reason; and 3) The use of time-worn, outmoded, insensitive and meaningless words. Imperfect words are the product of a color-blind memory and reason. This color blindness has a dominant influence on our spiritual and mental constitution, which is dependent upon our physiological constitution. Just as the function of a machine depends on its physical and mechanical construction, our mental and spiritual functions also depend greatly on our way of eating and drinking, which largely determine our physiological constitution.

Both the quality of our food and our way of eating have changed enormously over a period of thousands of years. In fact, eating and drinking, as well as our environment and way of living, have changed completely just in the last two thousand years. The human function of adaptability, of which reason and memory are only part, has also changed with the ages and with the changes of the human physiological constitution. Yet, we cannot return to the method of eating and the foods of two thousand or more years ago. We must create a new method of living, eating, and drinking that is appropriate to our own age and times. This is already long overdue.

But, before we can renew our way of life, it is necessary to renovate some of the outmoded and inappropriate definitions of words that we use for daily conversation and communication. This is much simpler and can be accomplished more easily and quickly than the physiological or dietetic revolution.

Happiness and 24 Other Important Words

There are one or two dozen very important words that must be brought up to date as soon as possible. Due to the misinterpretation of these words, we have repeatedly alternated between the completely futile and tragic comings and goings of peace and war for thousands and thousands of years. It will be very helpful to establish universal definitions for the following words:

freedom	motion	memory
justice	value	imagination
peace	human being	thought
happiness	fate	pleasure
love	reason	energy
truth	heart	wealth
kingdom of heaven	pleasure	matter
intuition	senses	adaptbility
mind	insight	will
conscience		

All of these words have both a relative and an absolute meaning, but I shall refrain from speaking about all of them except one;

that extremely important word is *happiness*. I shall speak of absolute happiness. The definition: Happiness is to accomplish all that one dreams (wishes), as much as one wishes, without depending on any tool or implement or help from others. The other happiness is that which is usually spoken of everywhere; what, then, is happiness in a relative sense? That is very simple to answer if one grasps the meaning of absolute happiness. Relative happiness (happiness of this world) is to accomplish what one wishes depending on various aids or tools and within the social circumstances of the age and times.

Absolute happiness is eternal and free, while the other is limited in time and space and is often ephemeral and illusory. Within the likes of a democratic society, in spite of careful thought and consideration for one another, still one may afflict another with a kind of happiness that is, in fact, the root of distress and sorrow for that person. Relative happiness can be purchased with money, authority, cleverness and trickery, knowledge, or ruthless sagacity. In other words, it may be gained through the use of a tool. On the other hand, happiness in the absolute sense can only be achieved through justice, and it causes neither pain nor sorrow to anyone. It is inexhaustible ,and its usefulness penetrates into every aspect of life. The achievement of this kind of happiness may seem impossible at first. But, if one truly grasps the compass of universal order, it is, different from Lockean liberty, within our power to actually embrace.

With this compass of judgment readily at hand and prepared for use, anyone can easily realize and maintain all relative forms of happiness as soon as they present themselves. You will have the potential to realize at will both relative and absolute happiness as well as anything else you desire. This compass is an instinctive biologically and physiologically precise tool of justice.

Jesus stated: "To he who has justice, it will be given in abundance, but to he who has not, it will be taken away from him even what he has." (Matthew 25:29)

In the time of Christ, the word *happiness* in the relative sense did not exist. This kind of happiness was called unhappiness. Indeed, it was Jesus himself who labeled it as such: "You see all this before you? Truly, I say unto you, there will not be left there one stone upon another that will not be thrown down." (Matthew 24:2) Here I will once again revive it anew. The word *happiness* degenerated from that time up to the present day. If your happiness cannot last for a long time, make no mistake about it, it is relative. Happiness limited either in time or space is nothing but unhappiness itself. If you were to inherit the throne of a king and you could do and have literally anything and everything that you wanted for a period of one, five, or even fifty years, and then in the end you were to be guillotined, would you call this happiness?

Jesus said, "For I tell you, unless your justice exceeds that of the Scribes and Pharisees, you will never enter the kingdom of heaven." (Matthew 5:20) The order of the universe, our compass, is the justice spoken of by Jesus. You must first possess it in order to enter the land of freedom and happiness. If you possess this compass and are able to wield it freely, you have already obtained the kingdom and you can accomplish whatever you choose for as long as you choose to do so. Now, perhaps, you can begin to see the true meaning and great importance of judo, for the essence of judo—adaptability—is the real compass of happiness.

Adaptability and the Essence of Judo

If you wish to learn judo, that is, to enter into a *dojo* and study the way of masters such as Kano and Ueshiba, you must change your view of life and become like a small child. If you can actually do this, you have not only realized the kingdom of heaven, but you are also already halfway towards becoming a master. You have already grasped the most important point. If you continue now, with this childlike, pure state of beginner's mind, to practice diligently and regularly, you will sooner or later gain mastery. The real problem is, how can you—without the aid of any exterior means or device—actually gain, and make a part of yourself, the fresh and wholesome adaptability of a strong, robust, and healthy child?

A little kitten has never gone into the school of judo, but, when it is unexpectedly thrown high into the air for the first time in its life by a mischievous child, it knows how to land with its four feet planted squarely on the earth. It knows judo! It is a born master! Indeed, all the animals, including humans, were originally like this. But education has stifled this marvelous adaptability in human beings. Judo is an art and method for reviving this spontaneous adaptability. When a kitten is just a kitten, when it is just born, it has a marvelous adaptability.

All the animals and all vegetables, including even microbes, lice, and fish of remarkable colors in the depths of the seas, have such marvelous adaptability. Giant bears living at the North Pole, sporting and delighting in their marvelous ability, regardless of burning heat or freezing temperatures of 30 or 40 degrees below zero, know nothing of human problems. They never sell their time for money or go off to become soldiers. They attack when necessary and defend themselves bravely and wisely. They are adventurous and risk their whole existence constantly, but they never imitate our stupidity, attempting to destroy their own species as we do with our inhuman bombs. They are much more polite and courteous than we are. The morality of the beasts is much more elevated than that of the human. The human is really a beast among beasts. There is much written about this in the books of Seton, the Fabre, and the Maeterlincks.[25]

What has become of human adaptability? Has it been lost? Fortunately not. It is, however, in a totally weakened and degenerated state. It often succumbs even to the attack of very adventurous and invisible microbes. These tiny microbes, who are able to kill this extraordinary giant—are they not great teachers of judo?

Jesus Christ, who fought alone against thousands of powerful enemies and, in the end, secured the most final and almost permanent victory, was a champion of judo. I will speak more of this in another chapter.

Napoleon was also a champion, although he had never learned the art that leads one to become an emperor. He lost the final battle because he placed too much confidence in his own power. Kant and Hegel, Marx and Lenin are also remarkable champions. So are Scott and Nansen.[26] Marx was the strongest, however, because he utilized the power based on the greatest of algebraic functions (distance/time) and minimized the time factor. Ralph Waldo Emerson, Henry David Thoreau, Abraham Lincoln, Benjamin Franklin, Jean Jacques Rousseau, George Bernard Shaw, Anatole France, and Romain Rolland were all great champions, and, yet, some among them died young. This indicates that they did not have time to practice physiological judo or that they were not especially interested in the preservation of health through proper nutrition or diet.

A Different Kind of Medicine

This is why I am telling you of a different medicine that is, in fact, nothing more than an application of the unique principle of the philosophy and science of the Far East. This will assist you greatly in perfecting your art and your comprehension of judo's technique and its underlying principle. Furthermore, it will enable you to enjoy practicing for as long as you choose.

My medicine is a physiological art or technique for the realization of the single most important quality, the superb character of a small child. It is, therefore, the key to the kingdom of heaven. It is a special art which revives one's enfeebled adaptability to become more like that of a kitten.

It is a different kind of medicine, totally unknown in the West until recently. It is an art of rejuvenation and long life, a medicine and dietetic regime that restores youthfulness and freedom. It is a study of health that makes us younger every day without the use of any special treatments or techniques. It is a blueprint for a happy and healthy life. It is extremely practical, simple, inexpensive, and easy to realize for anyone, anytime or anyplace. This medicine has a history of more than five thousand years. It is a physiological application of the dialectic principle of life, which has been totally ignored even in Japan since the importation of Western civilization about a century ago.

Let me here interject a small episode: At the beginning of World War II, there was one day, among the sick persons who came to see me, an invalid (tubercular and nephritic) named Keibu Hakozaki, 42 years of age, who had been bedridden for two years. He was a teacher of fencing (*kendo*) and held the grade of seventh *dan*. He was at the point of retiring completely from teaching due to this illness.

In two months, he was cured by my macrobiotic dietetic directions, which cost him nothing. He put aside all medicines and treatments and only ate some grains and certain vegetables. In fact, this diet relieved him a great deal financially as well. Some months later, he appeared at the *Butoku-kai* (fencing *dojo* in Tokyo) where he had previously taught. Upon invitation, he sparred with one of his seniors (*senpai*) of the eighth *dan*. The latter was amazed at the great progress his colleague had made during his two years in bed. How was this possible? It was actually a very simple matter. Due to his rejuvenated adaptability, he had become lighter and more rapid and sharp in his movement. Some months later, he was promoted to eighth *dan*. This is one among hundreds of miraculous cures.

Returning for a moment to the words listed earlier, what is the definition of love? To love in the absolute sense is to lead others, born in the midst of eternal happiness and yet unaware of its existence, to trade their insatiable attachment for worldly possessions and their incessant search for ephemeral and fleeting pleasures for the practical realization of eternal happiness. The most practical step towards this is the rejuvenation of our physiological constitution, which is, as we have seen, the foundation of absolute happiness and peace.

Chapter 9

From Health to Peace

We concluded in the preceding chapter that physiological health is the most important basis of happiness. It is the foundation of freedom and equality and, consequently, of democracy and peace.

There is a beautiful saying in Chinese philosophy, "If you desire world peace, you must first establish peace in the nation; if you wish to establish peace in the nation, you must first establish peace in the family; finally, if you desire to establish peace in the family, you must first of all establish physiological harmony and peace within yourself." In other words, you must establish your own physical and mental health.

This is the ethics of the Chinese and of the Far East. Thus, the ethics of the East is physiological and includes all philosophy, science, politics, economics, and education. It is the science of humanity, which was postulated by the democracy of Sir James Bryce[27] and the medicine of Dr. Alexis Carrel.[28]

If a democracy declines, this springs from the negligence of its physiological basis. If today's democracy does not run smoothly, it is most likely due to this same cause. If a nation rises in stature and flourishes, it is because that nation is built not only on a solid base but on a practical ideology as well. The Chinese study of health is steeped in ethics, and, at the same time, it is a technical and a practical philosophy. Philosophy and technique are inseparable. It is the synthesis of these two factors that creates the uniqueness of the Far East. Philosophy and science are fused into a single principle by the unique principle. It is because of this principle that China as well as

India, a much larger area than all of Europe, were in relative peace until the importation of Western civilization. Even the wars in China and India were not strategic wars, and Chinese strategy was a strategy of peace. In a word, the wars of the East, especially those of China, were ceremonious, picturesque, and sporting; there was neither cowardice nor great cruelty such as the use of the atomic bomb.

A state of physiological and moral health is the single most important unit in the establishment of peace in the daily life of the individual in society and in the world. A peace so established is concrete and lasting. Unfortunately, however, the way to apply this wonderful principle to the daily life of the individual is not at all explicitly pointed out. The religions of love, of loving and being loved, are one kind of art. They are a practical way of developing and refining one's physical, physiological, and moral adaptability. This adaptability calls forth the extremely important judgment of the instinct, which had previously been veiled by acquired knowledge. It is an art of becoming like little children.

Judo, as I have already mentioned, is the art of polishing and refining the adaptability of the instinct through practice. Adaptability is a passenger vessel constructed by nature so that those who cross the ocean of life may succeed regardless of any difficulties or great tempests. Religion is one kind of philosophical or spiritual technique for developing this adaptability, and judo is a kind of physical or athletic technique that teaches the same thing. From the first day of conception until our death, instinct is the most important pilot in our life.

Miyamoto Musashi, a great sword master of the 17th century who never attended any school or had any specific teacher, fought over fifty battles against opponents with live blades, and yet he was never defeated or injured even once. He had no teacher and yet, through training himself in the way of the sword and studying the unique principle, was able to develop his adaptability to the highest. He was a samurai who became a philosopher and at the same time a master sculptor, calligrapher, painter, architect, and poet. When one becomes really excellent in any school of the *do*, this ability and understanding becomes applicable to all facets of life. Musashi stated,

"The mentality of the way of martial strategy is nothing different from the mind of everyday routine life."[29]

Schools of the Dō

It is a curious thing that all the masters of the *do,* as well as the wise saints and scholars such as Jesus, Buddha, Confucius, Lao Tsu, Musashi, Mencius, and Kenshin Uesugi, do not speak to us in any detail concerning the conduct of life. They did not speak, much less write down, their philosophy for posterity. Rather, they were masters in actual practice. They had no desire to separate the principle from the practice by writing. This, in itself, is one great strength of the schools of the *do.* Masters of any of the schools of the *do* never write books or texts on the principles of their schools; often, it is forbidden. The deepest teachings (*okugi*) of the various schools of the *do* are always passed down only by oral teaching (*kuden*) from father to son or from the master to the highest student. This *kuden* is sometimes presented in the form of a very beautiful scroll on ornate paper. But what is found in this scroll is the name of the master and the student, the date, a list of the basics of that teaching (*do*), and sometimes a symbolic drawing, which no one can decipher except the student for whom it is destined. It is absolutely worthless to anyone else. No one else can judge the meaning of the secret teaching. Accordingly, the majority of ordinary teachers are unable to teach their students how to live their lives. They cannot attract or maintain students. Their schools, as well as their techniques, die. In this way, all of the schools of the *do* are relatively unproductive.

It is a very much criticized system, even ridiculed by educators today. Modern education or Western-style education is exactly the opposite of this; mass production is the axis on which it revolves. Thanks to this *kuden* system, however, all the various forms of Japanese fine arts, ancient philosophy, science, and technology have survived quite intact. The very highest-level arts and the principles underlying them have been passed down and maintained up to this present time including the dance, traditional medicine and nutrition, and haiku poetry, to mention just a few that have survived. Thanks to the many various schools of ancient tradition, the Goncourts were able to become aware of the great masters of *Ukiyo-e* painting, Hiroshige and Utamaro. Beautiful paintings and pottery by Sesshu, as well as beautiful kimono made by many unknown masters, have also been preserved.

The schools of the *do* never advertise or make propaganda. This is against the principle of the *do*. They hide their faces and are invisible, especially to strangers or the uninitiated. If there had been a Lafcadio Hearn for each school of the *do*, what great pleasure and happiness the whole world would have received. The *dojo* is essential for preserving the unique principle as a means of developing adaptability. It is not a place for the purpose of raising up idle dreamers or training people to be habitual copies of a master who in turn label themselves as self-styled masters.

I, myself, thanks to the poverty of my parents, did not attend school regularly and always maintained the primitive mentality that I infinitely adore. I am self-made and self-taught like Master Ueshiba, for whom I cherish a deep respect and affection.

One day, while speaking to a group of about thirty judges and attorneys, I was astonished in posing the following question to them: "What is the definition of a nation or a state?" Some of them responded with phrases borrowed from Western authors like Jellinek or Locke, but no one could answer me correctly.

At another conference, I posed this question to a group of about thirty high school teachers: "What is the most precious virtue in this world? Money, knowledge, honesty, power?" Finally, a very serious old professor of ethics said. "It is sincerity, I think."

"What is sincerity?" I asked.

No one could give the definition of sincerity, except in dictionary terms. Judges who do not know the definition of the state and teachers who do not know the meaning of sincerity, such are the fine specimens of school-made people or products of academic mass production in Japan. These are the academic leaders. It is, therefore, perfectly natural that societies with such leaders should carry on fratricidal wars, conflicts, deceit, or robbery in the beautiful name of justice, patriotism, political freedom, or socialism.

In the schools of the *do,* there are no Sundays or holidays. Learning how to live one's daily life is the purpose of this training. All these activities are done with liveliness and pleasure from morning until evening and sometimes even from evening until morning, 365 days a year. This is what is called *shugyo*—spiritual training in everyday life. It is very interesting, enjoyable, inexpensive, and productive. This school is open to everyone, everywhere, and yet those who are able to graduate from it are very few. From one point of view, we can say it is a school with seven Sundays a week, where there are no classes held. It is a kind of school of life where one also learns many technical skills.

The school of judo, the *dojo* (literally, the place of the way), is a building that has one main room in which there is nothing but the *tatami* mats that one practices on. The disciples are all boarders who do the cleaning, the gardening, and take care of all the daily and domestic affairs. It is truly a place for learning how to live. In the old days in Japan, these *dojos* were to be found nearly everywhere. Really superior *dojos* were few in number, and yet there were actually quite a few masters worthy of the title.

Today, there are many more public schools, but, in spite of enormous expenditures, there are few teachers who could assume the title of master or teacher of the way of life. Such schools are fine for creating slaves but can do little to prevent war. One could easily abolish all the public schools and governmental and private universities without causing a great deal of inconvenience, but one cannot and should not eliminate the schools of the *do.* They are a very rare, precious, and almost invisible existence, but that is all right; great masters and truly free people are also very rare. These schools offer an environment that brings our adaptability back to life and refines it still further. The places where one can physiologically refine one's adaptability have all but disappeared completely. It is difficult these days to accomplish it even in the schools of the *do.*

This is also why there are no really great people in Japan today. Even if there are some who appear to stand out as exceptional, the majority of them will no longer be mentioned after their death. They will be forgotten even before they reach the end of their lives. These people cannot be called great. From the point of view of human happiness, they are quite worthless. They are nothing more than manufacturers known for the production of reputable products, newspapers, or movies. They may have great value commercially, industrially, or in the world of sports or sensuality, but not for the real benefit of humanity.

One school that still remains as a forge of adaptability is the school of Zen (the Zen *dojo*). Unfortunately, there is not a single master of Zen today. The *dojos* of Zen are a little like the Catholic churches of today, void of soul.

The *do* is like a furnace that purifies the gold and silver and burns away the other useless materials. In the schools of the *do*, there is a rigid physiological selection that strains out those who do not have the appropriate qualities for becoming masters. It is an amazing contrivance or plan for the social development and progress of humanity as a whole.

Essential Point of the *Dojo*

The refinement of adaptability is primarily physiological, and this depends greatly on the daily food of the *dojo*. This is, in fact, the most essential point of the *dojo*. In all the Zen temples, as well as the Shinto shrines, the diet is still very rigorously practiced and is controlled by the most elevated disciples as a sacred tradition. Unfortunately, this is carried out today just as a tradition, and no one really grasps the deep significance of diet as it relates to the intuitive realization of the *dojo's* philosophy.

Furthermore, there is not even one judo *dojo* today that maintains the traditional macrobiotic dietary approach, which was the basis of health, happiness, and longevity in old Japan. The daily diet of a country is the true basis of a lasting culture, a living art, and a practical philosophy. It is this basis that gives that country and its individuals their own special characteristics. Without immersing oneself in the culture, art, philosophy, and especially the everyday life of a country as expressed through their eating habits, one can never hope to understand that country's culture.

There was a banker in Paris named Mr. H. His wife was a very pretty Japanese woman. He was very interested in Buddhism. After he retired from business, he would travel frequently to Japan for long visits to study the occult branch known as Shingon, the school of esoteric Buddhism. One day, he confessed to me that he could not understand Buddhism at all, in spite of his long studies.

"I suppose you have spent some years at the main temple of the Shingon sect at Mount Koya?"

"Yes, many years."

"And you lived in the temple?"

"Yes, always in the temple."

"Then you were fed in the Koya style of *shojin ryori*."

"Yes, yes, that's right."

"One hundred percent vegetarian style?"

"Exactly! Anything else is forbidden! It is rigorous Shingon." In that case, it is curious. I asked myself, if he ate completely in the vegetarian style of Buddhism, why was he unable to penetrate more deeply?

He continued: "But it was intolerable for me... One hundred percent vegetarianism. You can imagine, can't you?"

"Then?"

"Then, it was on Sundays that I escaped."

"You escaped from the temple! From the mountains? You descended?"

"Every Sunday, I descended. I rushed to Osaka to have my European meal at the Hotel Osaka and to spend a night in a European bed. Yes, I ate seven days' worth of meat in one evening. And then, Monday morning, I went back into the mountains."

"This is why you were unable to penetrate the depths of the more advanced teachings of Buddhism."

"What do you mean?"

"You studied Buddhism for many years. You have been to Japan many times for this purpose, but you left your body completely outside of Japan. Or rather, I should say, you have put your body in a one hundred percent Buddhist environment, but your whole interior environment was in Europe, nourished in the European style."

"But why not?"

"You have to nourish yourself in the Buddhist style if you want to comprehend Buddhism. It is a little bit like tasting a cake. If you would comprehend it, you have to study the composition, the confection, and the price. This will be sufficient in order to understand it from a peripheral view. To comprehend exactly what the cake is, however, you must taste it. You have to churn it around in your stomach and intestines and then let it be distributed to each of your cells where it can be burned up and changed into energy. In this way, you can discern and verify whether it is good to eat, whether it gives you strength or injures your health and diminishes your resistance some hours or days later. In this way, you can understand it completely. Abstract or conceptual comprehension by the brain alone is not complete, and to comprehend it with your stomach alone is also not sufficient. The same holds true for your cells. It must be understood with your whole existence—your conduct and activity; your society; your life itself. In other words, you must investigate everything from the most insignificant to the greatest, and then make this a part of your actual feeling and intuition. You must see from a view of justice.

"If you would comprehend Buddhism, you must place yourself right in the middle of the environment that has produced it. To love a single flower, you must love the whole plant: not only its stem, its leaves, its roots, but also its environment, its history, and its distant origin."

If you love the spirit of Christianity, you must comprehend it in its totality: its past, its origin, its founder, its history, its devotees, and its condition of life. Without practicing what Jesus practiced, you will not comprehend his spirit. He said, "Freely you have received, freely give." How many among you have understood and practiced this teaching?

If Jesus returned, would he call you Christians? Would he call you Pharisees, or would he call you pagan heretics? Would he call you Hebrew Scribes? Are you really, in fact, any of these? A moment ago, I spoke about the cake. It is in the likeness of that same meaning that I am asking you this question.

My Natural Medicine

Whether or not you are Christians is not the question here. The great question is whether you wish to comprehend only the judo or aikido that is in your brain, or that which depends on your complete and total environment. If you wish to comprehend it completely without suffering excessive physical difficulty and also without taking a great deal of time, you must observe at least these simple recommendations that I offer you now. This is only one part of my natural medicine, but I offer it to you freely:

1. Do not eat too much yin (expansive) food, that which diminishes or neutralizes the sodium content in your body. In a word, take only small amounts of water, very little fruit, little salad.

2. Do not take anything that damages your basic physical quality or destroys your energy—for example: vinegar, all sugary foods, nightshades, coffee, chocolate or pastries, soft drinks—for a period of at least one month.

3. Brown rice, millet, buckwheat, and all the various unrefined grains should constitute at least 50 percent of your total diet.

That is all. It is very simple, and yet it will guarantee you a big step on the way to self-improvement—good health, prevention of illness, and the preservation of your youthfulness. This is the unknown and very simple medicine completely simplified for your practice. Try it for one month. You will already be able to verify the results. It is a part of the dietary regimen in all of the original traditional schools of the *do*. At the same time, it is the first practical lesson for curing all present or future illness by means of my macrobiotic method. And it costs you almost nothing.

Meats, animal protein, butter, cheese, fish, animal fat, and all animal products are completely unnecessary for maintaining your health; these products, as well as all other manufactured and modern industrial products, may be abolished completely from your daily diet in order to reestablish or stabilize your physical condition and to develop and fortify your adaptability, imagination, memory, and judgment.

Due to your modern, scientific, Western knowledge, you are somewhat hindered in your ability to understand the importance of these preparatory remarks, and, yet unfortunately, I cannot take time to give you a detailed explanation here. My method dates back at least five thousand years. It is based on the primitive mentality (so named by my dear colleague, the late Lévy-Bruhl), and, at the same time, it is directly derived from the philosophical matrix of the three great religions. It would be necessary to speak of it at great length here in order to study it deeply; but this book is not devoted to that purpose, and you are not philosophers or specialized dieticians.

These words of caution are a very important gift, and I give them to you as a present from my heart. They are the results of my clinical studies and practice of nearly forty years. I have guided more than 150,000 ill persons back to health by this natural medicine, in Japan as well as in Europe. Some of them attended my clinic directly, while others were influenced through courses in traditional medicine at my institute. Many, especially in France and other European countries, first came into contact with me through correspondence or through my publications. For nearly twenty years, I have not returned to France, where I spent thirteen years in all since my first visit in 1914.

Finally, I have settled in Japan. I have been very much occupied with my patients, among whom there are princes and princesses, generals, professors, and doctors. I have aimed at the rebirth of all the ancient schools of the *do*, especially medicine and the unique principle of Eastern philosophy. I have presided over the research for a new Japanese culture.

For three years, I was occupied with launching a movement for a World Federation or World Government in Japan and the establishment of its theoretical constitution (discussed in later chapters). To this end I translated Professor Northrop's *The Meeting of East and West* into Japanese. I also translated Alexis Carrel's *Man, the Unknown* and others from French to Japanese. Since World War II,

I have founded four monthly publications: *Health; The Compass; World Government; and the International Compass.* This work has kept me from giving health consultations, and for three years I have stopped seeing sick people, except for very difficult and grave cases.

Also within my credentials is the effectiveness of my method against the effects of atomic radiation. In Nagasaki, at the epicenter of the atomic bomb explosion, there were two hospitals—the hospital annexed to the University of Nagasaki, and that of the Catholic monastery. In the first, the majority (more than 80 percent) of all patients, doctors, professors, students, and nurses died quickly or within two months following the blast. In the Catholic hospital, there was not a single death. The director, Dr. Akizuki, is one of my disciples; he and many others were saved by macrobiotics. How this was possible is revealed in Dr. Akizuki's book.[30]

I have asked you to observe, for one month, my fundamental and preparatory suggestions in order that you might understand the underlying principles of judo or aikido, which, up to this time, have never been explained in writing by anyone. I wonder if this experience will suffice for you. If you can really understand, there would be no greater happiness for me.

Chapter 7

The Eternal Peace of Jesus

Jesus was one great master of judo. He was attacked by thousands of enemies who were much more powerful, and yet he conquered them and his victory has lasted nineteen centuries. The Pharisees, the Scribes, the heretics, and all those who came after his death respected Jesus even though they were unable to understand him. Even this generation of vipers—the unhappy people of today who are enchained by discouragement and anxiety—has been forced to respect him and his works.

Jesus never used force. He forgave his enemies even when they tried to kill him. He utilized their power against them until finally in the end, they killed him. In spite of that, it is his enemies who, for nineteen hundred years, have been unhappy and punished by being exposed on the cross of the people's judgment. Jesus, on the other hand, is loved by the people for his nonresistance, nonviolence, and his effortless power. He has been able to give courage, pleasure, peace, nobility, eternity, and tranquillity to the great majority of the people for nineteen hundred years, even after his death. His enemies have had only sadness, remorse, hatred, and despair. Who is the conqueror? Jesus, the distributor of eternal joy, peace, happiness, and courage—or his enemies, the generators of hatred, remorse, and sadness? Jesus is eternal peace while his enemies represent anxiety and fear.

"The supreme method is to obtain victory by apparent defeat." These are the words of Sun Tsu. Could this not describe or represent the spirit and deeds of Jesus?

Fear, remorse, hatred, and sadness are the emotions that rule the vanquished. That which gives joy, peace, serenity, and courage is victory. This is the eternal victory of Jesus.

Judo is the way of Jesus. When two forces of opposite direction collide, combat or conflict is born. This develops in two different ways depending on the proportion of yin and yang components.

- The yang, developed by power and training, serves as a fortress.
- The yin, developed through spiritual searching, creates adaptability.

The yang fortress, created by power and hard training, is very limited by the laws of physiology and biology; while the method of battle, depending on spiritual searching, develops more and more. It is divided into two new directions: Weapons (yang) and Strategy (yin). Weapons are of various kinds, and they range from a simple stick or stone (yang) to firearms, among which the atomic bomb (yin) is the newest. Weapons all fall under the category of force (yang).

Strategy also develops in two new directions: The yang type ranges from the simple maneuver to the very complicated strategy of Lenin, and the yin variety is much less visible and more spiritual, ranging from espionage to the philosophical strategy of Sun Tsu. Sun Tsu's strategy was aikido rather than judo; it is continuing to develop even now. Its supreme pinnacle is the strategy of Jesus Christ. In this sense, *aiki* is another narrow gate that leads you to the country of life, the kingdom of heaven, or, in other words, to the universal country of peace and freedom.

Whether one enters by the narrow gate of Christianity or by another way, the important thing is to gain understanding and put it into practice for the development of your physiological adaptability. This is why most people cannot find the narrow gate and believe that it is foolish to seek it. They are unaware of how to make use of their eyes and their ears so that real seeing, hearing, and understanding can become a possibility. Otherwise, how can we obtain the powers of reason and comprehension, memory and judgment?

If you do not have these marvellous qualities of instinct, you have only to restore your physiological constitution. Without this, all is impossible for you.

Faith

Jesus said: "If you have faith and do not doubt, you shall say unto this mountain, be thou removed and cast into the sea, and it shall be done." (Matthew 21:21)

Here I have the pleasure, as a primitive man born in the East and, as of yet, untouched by the Western spirit, of interpreting for you this word, *faith*. Faith means the spiritual quality of a small and very happy child. It is the state of mind of the kingdom of heaven, which knows nothing of human laws or morals. In Japanese, it is called *shin,* and it means something completely different from the term called *faith* in modern Western language. This situation is the same for the words *respect, chastity, human being,* and *freedom,* as well as the two dozen most fundamental and important words I set forth earlier.

The word *faith* (creed or belief) of the West appears to correspond with the Japanese word *shin* or *makoto*, but in the philosophical sense, unless I am completely mistaken, it is quite the opposite.

Faith, the supreme integral wisdom, has a quality that is totally transparent, with the power to permeate all things. In outward appearance, it is elegant, graceful, and full of joy. Thus, the faith called *shin* is not credo or belief; it is complete wisdom or understanding of truth. In essence, it is justice or freedom; in appearance, it is love and joy. Let me explain it in a parable: Faith is an ocean of wisdom with neither surface nor floor, without end in either space or time, and yet all is in perfect order. There is not one infinitesimal particle, even of infinite speed, that is working outside of this universal solidarity. Because of its great speed and the ultra-transparency of its constitution, nothing can be detected by sight or sense in this ocean but elegantly dancing myriads of pearls like bubbles of joy, moving spirally in all directions.

The faith of the Far East is a resonance produced in the individual (small self) by the greatest individuality (large self, the infinite universe); it is not an illusory connection or a fleeting communication between one individual and another.

Many people, curiously enough, believe that the seat of thought, imagination, and the mind encompassed by our memory are found in our brain. Actually, this is somewhat reversed. Our body, especially our brain, is an instrument like a radio receiver that automatically picks up any frequency. This automatic quality itself is that which is known as memory, thought, and imagination. Thus, our small brain is like a connection to the large "brain" of the universe itself. These things, as well as the powers of reasoning and will, are not merely a receiver that picks up radio waves; they are like a very advanced and sensitive television set that operates in time—in the past, the present, and the future. Within our brain alone, there are at least ten billion vacuum tubes called cells. Our body is soaked in the depths of the infinite undulating ocean of the pre-electronic waves of mind, soul, or spirit. Our thinking mind is not contained within this fragile and ephemeral prison of the body, quite the contrary. For this very reason, we are able to think, imagine, memorize, compare one scene with another.

Our body is immersed to the marrow of our bones in the ocean of super high-speed electronic waves over the earth that are constantly passing through us. The speed of the earth's rotation around the sun plus the speed of the sun also moving around the Milky Way galaxy, combined with the movement of our earth as it also spins on its own axis while receiving this influence, equals a tremendous speed. Every instant, every second, our actions here on this earth are projected at this ultra-super speed into the far reaches of space. It is like a scene from a movie. At first, it is all rolled up and put away within the film case, but when it becomes extended through the lens of the miraculous extrasensory projector of our mind and realized on the screen of our consciousness, we are able to witness all the variety of life's scenes every moment and from any place. This is certainly the most complicated of all projectors.

Faith, like that of Jesus, is the strength and the mechanism behind such a mind. This miraculous projector projects scenes one after another in front of its lens at a tremendous speed. Furthermore, it is able to select and magnify any part of any scene, even one that has already been rolled up and put away, completely at its own discretion. Indeed, it is the multi-origin projector of all scenes. At the same time, it is also the light that illuminates them whenever we want to view them. It is the film, the playwright, the set designer, the scene painter, the orchestra, the conductor, the cameraman, the producer, the actors, and even the paying spectators. It writes, produces, and projects as it wishes. The mind is the one infinite ocean of life, while physical bodies are infinitely numerous.

Physical bodies appear and fade away again like the foam on the ocean tide. But their Creator brings them forth and distinguishes them one from the other, and this allows us to establish understanding between ourselves. It is also the very reason why we tend to personify all other existences as well and treat them as if they were human. Such an attitude is not total ignorance. It is not blind faith or the attitude of a beggar who, with tears in his eyes, pleads for the grace of the Divine Creator. God is also unnecessary. We are ephemeral and illusory foam, physiologically speaking, but at the same time—because we have mind and feeling—we are also the creator of that infinite ocean of mind. Each of us contains this two-sided dialectic constitution. Therefore, even within the same individual, there is a constant conflict of body and soul (heart and mind), and this, of course, is prevalent among the greater majority of people.

Complementary Opposites and Antagonisms

This battle between the body and the soul changes into the following kinds of conflicts: The conflict between religion (spirit and soul) and science (sensory and, therefore, physical), and conflicts between the people in northern areas and the people of the South. The people of the North are accustomed to the permanent struggle for survival. They lack raw materials, natural resources, heat, and light while the southern peoples have easy access to light, heat, and nourishment. If anything, the southern people are too fortunate in this sense. This is why there are fortresses and long walls running from east to west like the Great Wall of China as well as three or four others that existed in England, northern Italy, and in the land of the Incas. These walls existed to defend the southern peoples against invasion from the North.

The northern people are in search of the plentiful raw materials, food supplies, and comfort existing abundantly in the South. In comparison, the inhabitants of the South are in need of protection against heat and light. Like most of the Buddhas, they spend their time discovering the secrets of Nirvana and the Vedantas.

There are still more examples, but I would like to refer you to the work of Ellsworth Huntington, *Civilization and Climate*.[31] In "Season of Birth," one of the chapters of this book, you will find different personality characteristics considered according to the season or month of birth in a given climate or locality. This is interesting, but the professor does not give a physiological explanation of individual character. Rather, he leaves us in mystery, declaring that if there are many top generals or soldiers among those born in the month of March, perhaps it is due to Mars, the god of war.

This is, however, completely off the mark. Those born in March, April, or May passed the last six months of their embryological period in the cold season. Their mothers, in order to keep warm and to balance the yin foods (which neutralize salts) taken in the earlier hot months of pregnancy, had to eat more yang foods rich in sodium. The last half of the embryological period is more important than the first from the point of view of our physiological constitution. Furthermore, there are mostly yang foods available during the yin season, and it is necessary, therefore, to eat more salty foods regardless of one's personal preference. This is why those born in March are yang. In addition, there are many other conditions that govern, mold, and make up our total constitution. It should also be obvious that these various conditions all become opposite in countries south of the equator.

Opposites in time and space share mutual affinities and attraction. This is a partial expression of universal law in the physical as well as the physiological and psychological worlds. Such factors as heat and cold, male and female, and north and south do not influence us so directly as they do through the vegetables, grains, and other products produced in a given season and climate. These products form and stabilize our constitution. In essence, our daily diet is the main factor. The most important factor is how we choose, combine, prepare, and season our food. Of course, other important factors are how much and in what manner we eat.

Opposites are a curious thing, whether in space or time. Northerners and Southerners or those born in orbital antipodes (about six months apart) are very much attracted to one another. For example: Charles and John Wesley (December 18, 1707, and June 17,1729); Marx and Engels (May 5,1818, and September 28,1820); Lenin and Stalin (April 10,1870, and November 28,1879).

If they are too strongly attracted, a collision is produced. This is often seen when one or both people's judgment—world or universal concept—is on a low level or when they are coming from a narrow point of view based on preconceived ideas. If their object is money or land, of which there is only a certain amount available, it is very natural that they may run head-on into each other in brutal and often cruel dispute. On the other hand, if they have high judgment and a clear concept of world and universal reality, if they are able to rise above time and space and contemplate their differences objectively, then they will never reach the point of actual conflict. In a sense, the ultimate aim of judo and all the martial ways is to avoid this point, and the same can be said of Jesus's teachings.

The origins of disputes and conflicts inevitably arise from differences in our concept of reality, the world, and the universe. We each have different physiological constitutions, activities, and tendencies and our concept of the world is, more or less, eclipsed according to the surroundings of our embryological and infant life. Even in the case of identical twins, it is impossible to have all the same conditions embryologically, biologically, economically, politically, and sensorially. Thus, from the point of physiology and individual feeling, it is impossible to have the same image of the universe; according to physiological constitution, each person necessarily has a different way of seeing everything. Yet nothing is easier than to cherish the same reality of life from the extrasensory standpoint of mind, heart, or spirit. In any case, when there is an antagonism or conflict, it is in this place alone that two people can establish mutual understanding. For this purpose, a tiny tool like a switch, a key, or a formula will be sufficient: that is, a mapped-out diagram or intuitive grasp of universal order. This is the only valid compass in our everyday life.

A New Interpretation of Jesus's Teachings

It is necessary that the conflict or antagonism of opposite factors always exists everywhere, universally, in order to establish supreme peace, eternal and worldwide. We have the key that constantly mends and compensates for all antagonisms, changing them into complementary factors. That is the dialectic compass. It is reflected in the words of Jesus, but they are so outdated that it is difficult to correctly interpret their meaning. We are pursued by the need for a new edition of these words.

Aikido is actually an interpretation of Jesus's teachings, and this small book (as well as all of my other works) form a new edition of his teachings interpreted through the unique principle.

Jesus said, "Yes, look at it all. Truly I tell you, not one stone will be left upon another, they will all be thrown down." (Matthew 242)

Also: "Take care that no one misleads you. For many will come claiming my name and saying, 'I am the Messiah,' and many will be misled by them. The time is coming when you will hear of wars and rumor of wars. See that you are not alarmed. Such things are bound to happen; the end is yet to come. For nation will go to war against nation, kingdom against kingdom; there will be famines and earthquakes in many places. All these things are the first birthpangs of the new age. You will be handed over for punishment and execution; all nations will hate you for your allegiance to me. At that time, many will fall from their faith, they will betray one another and hate one another." (Matthew 24:10)

Today we hear the rumors of war approaching closer all the time. We hear people crying out, "Take care... not one stone will be left upon another..."

All things that are the product of our own sense data—our precious bodies, our families, our parents—are passing and will never be able to be replaced once they are gone. Why then, for God's sake, do we insist on working ourselves into a delirious frenzy and running at breakneck speed towards our own destruction and decomposition? Is it perhaps too much for me to suggest that it is because we do not know the true spirit of judo?

There are today, even among Christians and Buddhists, those who charm the masses, saying, "I have a plan for resolving all the problems of life, a plan that will save humanity," or indeed, "I have invented a super nuclear bomb that will destroy all your enemies where they stand, instantaneously." These so-called Christians or Buddhists may incite some people—the ignorant majority, empty-minded after the fashion of Zen—and yet they themselves never realize anything. They are Christians and Buddhists on paper alone. They are imitation fortune-tellers, if not mere portraits.

In this way, these false Christians and Buddhists are the real Pharisees, the Scribes, and the heretics. But your father in heaven knows what you have need of. So seek first harmony and the kingdom of heaven, principle 7 of the order of the universe (see Chapter 7), and its justice, principles 1 through 6, and all else will be given unto you.

Chapter 11

World Government
of the People

The idea of a government of the people, by the people, and for the people was born some two hundred years ago in France. It increased and sent forth a light to establish a new civilization in Europe and America. All the institutions of old were overturned, and this idea dominated the Western World. The West, however, is always in conflict and suffocating from fear. It would really be beautiful if this new idea, born in the West, could be effective in saving the world from the chaos it has fallen into.

But what is Europe or the West? For the primitive mentality of the Far East, it is not another world at all but only a small peninsula at the western edge of the Eurasian continent. America is only a colony that was invaded by Europe. The peninsula called Europe has been nourished for some twenty-five hundred years by the ideas and concepts of its mother continent, Asia. The foundation of Western civilization is one of the many bibles of Asia; many elements of Eastern civilization were imported and translated by Western people such as the Greeks or Eastern Europeans and, later, the Romans. These Westerners changed the format of Asian civilization completely and turned it into utter chaos. In the eyes of the Orient, however, the changes that were made in the original works were simple, surface, and accepted at face value as being nothing more than of a mystical nature.

Complications arose from the difference between the Eastern and the Western mentality, both of which are extremes. Western mentality is a yang, masculine mentality while the Eastern might be christened as the yin spirit of the feminine mind. They are, therefore, exact opposites. Their respective climates and environments are also opposites. Yin mentality is born in a yang country under the influence of a yang climate. The reason for this is simply that a yang country or yang (hot) season allows mainly for the existence and abundant growth of yin grains and vegetables. A yang spirit, on the other hand, is born and nurtured in a yin environment where there are mainly yang grains and vegetables for life and growth. This is the dialectical constitution-order of the world and the universe and applies equally to all products and phenomena that are born within this world.

Because antagonisms exist everywhere on all levels, so do these two antagonistic mentalities also coexist everywhere in both East and West. Just as with day and night, summer and winter, or north and south, the balance between all antagonistic factors is only a matter of the ratio between the two essential factors of yin and yang. Such thinkers as Swedenborg, Dilthey, Driesch, Du Bois-Raymond, and William James, who tend towards the intuitive, mystical, and the spiritual or religious, actually have their orientation more in the East in spite of the fact that they are Westerners. In contrast to these people, there are such men as Confucius, Democritus, and others whose thinking is actually more Western, moralistic, mechanistic, or materialistic. The extremes of these two mentalities overlap and infiltrate each other, forming a new mentality altogether.

Prior to the Meiji Restoration, all of the revolutionary and military leaders of Japan were samurai, descendants of the most noble families of feudal times. They had the greatest pride in their own culture and traditions. These leaders took upon themselves the extremely difficult task of bringing a sense of intimacy with Western civilization to the minds and hearts of the people. The antagonistic extremes, East and West, are naturally drawn to each other and exert their respective influences.

As verified in the words of Spengler and Karl Jaspers, the greatest atrocities and crimes in history have been committed in Europe
or the West. This has caused the whole world considerable misery,
uncertainty, and anxiety. The West has led the world towards the
ruin and destruction we now experience as scientific and mechanical
civilization. This crisis was anticipated more than fifty years ago by
Nietzsche and Kierkegaard. Edward Carpenter[32] made a precise ac-
cusation concerning it as did Thoreau. Kou-hounming also criticized
it more severely. Tagore and Sorokin, Lin Yutang, and a good many
others anticipated it. Alexis Carrel gave warning of it, and Jacques
Maritain and Lecomte de Nouys lamented it.

But as Dostoevsky, Jaspers, and many others have said, this crisis, this disorder and destiny of civilization, was led by the spirit of
Christianity and accelerated by mechanical inventions that led to extremes by the instinct of the masses. This is the destiny of all that is
found in the relative, dialectical world. Westerners, however, having
not yet grasped this dialectical nature in their everyday life, continue
to torture themselves, striving in vain to become free of moral, cultural, economic, and political misery. They have invented two paths
of escape, both of which are, in themselves, dialectical dilemmas:

1. The colonization of the unexploited world of yin and primitive
Eastern peoples. First of all, in order to console or excuse themselves,
they invade while brandishing their Bibles, originally of Eastern origin. Then, with the use of yang and forcible methods, they enslave
the innocent, ignorant, honest, and weak people. This itself is the
destiny of Western civilization. It is like the son of Laius, abandoned
from birth on Mt. Cithaeron, taken in by merchants and fed in Western style in contrast to the vegetarians and farming people of the
East. He soon became full of curiosity, suspicious and doubtful of
everyone and everything. He also became large and full of brawn.
He then devised a means of using his strength combined with his
reason. He used scientific methods through which he was able to
eliminate everything that stood in his way. He killed his father, who
was an Eastern leader, and married his mother. He preached the philosophy of peace (monopolizing Christianity) and finally, in the end,

he tore out his own eyes. He could no longer see the world, much less the order of the universe. Behold the sad portrait of Oedipus under a modem pseudonym: Europe; the West; science.

2. The invention of machines. Machines create illusory wealth and abundance, which obscures vision and prevents perception of the order of the universe. The increase of sense data only furthers this insanity until the intensity of our own fortification leads us to self-destruction with atomic bombs.

We succeeded very well with our first method. The founding of the United States is the greatest example of that. The second method, however, has turned all the pleasure and successes of humanity into misery, desperate commercial and industrial competition, both hot and cold war, world anxiety, as well as various other threats and dangers within society. Because the European or Western emancipation of humanity has utilized these two methods, we are surrounded by catastrophe. This marks the death of modem civilization.

A World Government

However, the West is gradually awakening. It has realized the seriousness of its crime, the greatest homicide in human history. In order to redeem itself, it has discovered two new plans: 1) To establish a world government either by reforming or strengthening the United Nations or by creating a new world organization, and 2) To eradicate both communism and capitalism or to establish a new empire or utopia; to abolish Western civilization itself and prohibit its very powerful implement called science.

Both methods have the same goal: World peace and a society in which everyone is happy and free. For this purpose, certain minorities are now diligently researching a new formula for a world constitution. Meanwhile, the majority continues to pursue catastrophic strategy. This majority wants the abolition of Christianity, the annihilation of all past social institutions, peace by miracles, the protection of atomic bombs, and the advancement of science as a new religion.

From the point of view of Oriental philosophy, these efforts are

very courageous and admirable, but not necessary or useful. They
are somewhat after-the-fact or secondary solutions. Christianity, the
foundation of Western civilization, is actually firm and solid though
we may become slightly agitated with its superstructure. Its application is precise and, as a technique that deals with both the physically
manifest as well as the world of thought, it is truly wonderful. What
is necessary, however, is to revise the Bible in a way that has been
unknown until now. This new edition would contain a commentary
on primitive mind and spirit written by a primitive. The Oriental person today, who could actually qualify to write this, is extremely rare.
The essential qualification would be a primitive mind unscathed and
intact. The Bible, full of Greek modifications and Roman complications, has not been revised for over nineteen hundred years.

And there is no need to blame scientific technique. Unfortunately, science utilizes its means of exactness and precision only to study
certain realities and facts that belong to the realm of sense data, but
not at all to study what constitutes thought or contemplation. Science has little to do with the spiritual world, treating it superficially
at best. It deals solely with Western mentality and has little interest
in the phenomena of the East such as contemplation. Science does
not know what thought, memory, and contemplation are, and it is
especially ignorant concerning the mechanism behind these functions. Science has not as yet researched these areas, or perhaps it has
not yet developed sufficiently to handle these mechanisms. There is
a great deal of talk about the subconscious mind, but no one really
knows what it is. The same is true of thought, memory, peace, justice, freedom, the will, virtue, truth, energy, a monad, and instinct. If
science were able to elucidate the mechanism of thought, the means
of direct communication between God and humankind would be
opened, and virtually all things in this life would progress smoothly
from that point forward.

I tell you there are two new techniques that must be realized at
the same time in order to establish a free and peaceful world:

- To consolidate and fortify exact and precise knowledge

of our existence as well as facts or impressions gathered through the senses (sense data) by means of a compass that, continually and in all places, indicates the direction of peace and freedom for all of humanity.

- To elucidate the mechanisms of thought, memory, and contemplation. This is, in itself, the establishment of an absolute determinism (the order of the universe).

Knowledge of our existence and the facts just mentioned belong to our limited, relative world: in contrast, that which elucidates the mechanisms of thought, memory, and contemplation is the foundation of all knowledge. It is the constitution and order of the absolute infinite universe. The apparent antagonism of modem knowledge towards memory, instinct, and intuition necessitates another Cartesian revolution. One must undo all modern, scholastic knowledge and opinions. All of modern science and philosophy has become scholastic, outmoded, or even archaic.

A New Theory of Polarizable Monism

Herein lies the necessity for a new theory of polarizable monism—a unique and matchless worldwide, universal, spiritual, and intuitive sense of reality. We need a completely new method. It must be practical, but never dualistic.

Unless scientific knowledge has practical usefulness, it is meaningless. An intuitive sense of the world and the universe, of spiritual reality, including the mechanisms of memory and contemplation, is extremely important. It is fundamental and makes knowledge concrete. The research of scientific knowledge is indirect, secondary, and, moreover, illusory; that is to say, it never arrives at its goal. It is forever incomplete. Basic and primary research, of which our relative material existence is but an infinitesimal point, is direct. It requires and allows no intermediary or instrument to cloud the human intuition. It has already been cultivated and brought to perfection thousands of years ago by the great Eastern philosophers (or rather we should say people of wisdom) of ancient times (Lao Tsu, Buddha, and Jesus) who were known as saints and sages. Recently, in the West, this realm has been researched by Locke, Hegel, and Kierkegaard, although in a more or less incomplete manner. Science, on the other hand, under the influence of such learned men as Lavoisier and Newton, has developed with giant strides in the last two hundred years of Western history. Recently, in the East, there have been valiant efforts by Yukawa, H. Nagaoka, Tomonaga, and Sagane. Nevertheless, Far Eastern people are still far inferior and incomparably behind in scientific research. Each has his own speciality and takes special pride in it.

Science as a whole, however, is still only in its initial stages. It must be led and brought up properly by its mother, the spirit or mentality of the Orient. We are in a situation where science cannot yet even sufficiently understand the mother's words. An interpreter is needed. Here is the *raison d'etre* of the practical dialectic, a new method, the order of the universe, which expresses itself in the very simple and universal language of yin and yang. It is the direct language of the instinct, which everyone possesses from before their own birth. Mahayana Buddhism, Christianity, Islam, and the *tao* of Lao Tsu are only different interpretations of this language and are, for the most part, relatively inaccurate. Past interpretations are far too outdated for this modem age. The theories of Democritus or Heraclitus are good examples of poor and awkward attempts at interpreting it. The order of the universe is the basis of peace and freedom. It is an intuitive, universal view.

Modem scholars and philosophers of the West such as Jaspers, the Greek editors, the Roman complicators, and the mystical Europeans with their oversimplified commentary have this to say: Complete freedom will never be established on the earth. Freedom is the suppressing of our own whimsical, selfish, and egotistical desires. It is the eternal path beset with countless obstacles and difficulties, which people must continually dodge in order to reach happiness. History will never reach perfection. It eternally repeats the same things over and over again. It does not give us a single law that we can exalt or live our lives in accordance with. The same is true for the efforts of science. Humanity is destined to be forever unhappy.

The above is the fate of modern man's scholarship. Science ends in a new stoicism or scholasticism. Western civilization, which ventured forth with the goal of realizing all humanistic goals and dreams, has ended in a reactionary stoicism. In this world, everything that has a beginning eventually comes to an end, and beginning and end are always opposites; this is the first of the seven universal and eternal laws. Even if people accept facts, sense data, and the elements of existence at face value and distill them into authoritative laws, I still cannot accept their explanations when they are inevitably engulfed in the mentality of *credo quia absurdum est* ("I believe it because it is absurd").

I suggest that, as you have accepted Christianity for some seventeen hundred years, you now also attempt to accept a unique and matchless new method of elucidating the mechanisms of thought and memory simply and directly. This new method takes into consideration not only Western but also Eastern thought. I suggest that you place this new method in a position of high importance, even above that of your past beliefs. This would not cost even a billionth as much as today's scientific research on the murderous weapons of war.

The ancient thinkers, and particularly the Oriental meditators, arrived at the final end of thought, contemplation, and memory thousands of years ago. This final goal is the principle within all other principles, an intuitive sense of the world and the universe. All you have to do, however, is to practice the first simple lesson, the macrobiotic approach to correct diet. If you feel a great need to comprehend the primitive mind or Far Eastern philosophy and enter immediately into the heavenly kingdom of eternal peace and freedom, then, rather than study a lot of grandiose theory that you will likely not really comprehend, you can learn through actual training in judo or aikido to make a real and intuitive understanding of the way, the *do* or *tao*, an integral part of your own being. The first lesson is not very complicated, but it is extremely practical. It is the practice of yoga, simplified for everyone and especially for Westerners.

Above all and as soon as possible, enter into this heavenly kingdom. The door stands open wide; it is the assembly of peoples for world government. This is the building of Noah's ark. This ark will inevitably preserve those who will become the ancestors of our future race, the couples (yin and yang) of the future, from the flood (the baptism with fire and nuclear weapons). These survivors will be capable of founding a new human race. All the other animals and plants have already boarded. The new flood will come to destroy the whole world—universal inundation by tides, fire, machinery, and nuclear bombs. What we see everywhere on this planet is the beginning of torrential rains and floods of fire, of death and evil. We are in the presence of devils who are desperately occupied in the mass production of wars and nuclear weapons of total annihilation.

Let us embark!

Climb into the new Noah's Ark christened *The World Government*. It is raining fire and evil everywhere. Make haste. Let us return to the biblical cottage of the *tao*, the order of the universe. Can't you hear the tremendous roar of the bombs falling? There are great winds and lightning flashes. The only reception you receive on the radio by your side is static noise.

You Can Create Miracles

If you really have the desire to do so, you can create a peaceful world any time you decide. By seeing all things through the lens of the order of the universe, you receive the ability of miracles—the power of understanding, creative imagination, recollection, thought, and the ability to shed tears for those who are less fortunate than yourself—from the Universal Proprietor. As a result, nothing is impossible for you.

The Gentiles, the Pharisees, and the Heretics fought tooth and nail for food, clothing, and shelter, but do not be overly concerned with these things. Such pursuits are of little value in establishing world peace and harmony, much less individual peace. This is because these things spoil and disappear instantly. They cannot be maintained and, when we pass into the next world, we must leave them all behind. To spend our efforts for the accumulation of such things is of no avail; it is all in vain. Life is too short to be spent for worldly possessions when work of a much higher nature will suffice to meet all our immediate needs. This world is too small to be only concerned with private businesses, the amassing of knowledge or possessions, sexual pleasure, the attachment to children, authority, or any of the things that last only one-millionth of a second in the great-grandfather clock of universal time.

Now you have become aware of the dialectical order-constitution of the universe; you have the compass that always and everywhere indicates the way towards health and freedom, happiness and peace. Now you must go forth and cure the sick, those who have lost their power of will; revive the dead, all those who cannot establish freedom and happiness; save the mental and physical lepers, the spiritually blind who have no memory, imagination, judgment, or common sense, the incurable ones who are unable to change the direction of their own lives; and cast out the demons, those who seek only momentary pleasures and the amassing of ephemeral possessions.

Chapter 12

A World in Peace
and Freedom

Japan was defeated. It was demolished, crushed, and vanquished. This is too bad for imperialist Japan, but it is just fine for the real Japan, which is based on an eternal principle. Imperialist Japan substituted the Western style for all the traditional institutions and educational systems of the *do*. For this reason, it collapsed. I predicted World War II in 1930 and criticized Japanese militarism very severely after that time. I also predicted the unprecedented defeat of Japan twelve months before the attack on Pearl Harbor, just as I had predicted the cruel assassination of Gandhi five years before his death.

All this, of course, ended in the prohibition and later the confiscation of my publications. Finally, I myself was also put into prison. Twenty years ago, I could feel the oncoming and inevitable defeat of Japan and had hoped to destroy and sweep away the rootless sprout that Japan had become. It was trying to destroy its own parental tradition and all the schools of the *do* with the borrowed strength of Western civilization. This militaristic Japan was crushed and scattered. The two atomic bombs dropped on the cities of Nagasaki and Hiroshima tragically killed 313,884 innocent souls. They were dead where they stood. This must have cost the United States a great deal of money. If they had been a little wiser, they would have avoided the loss. They had only to give, in order to help the poverty of Japan, a thousandth of the sum of money that was spent on the war. Or, if they chose not to give anything at all, they need not have spent even one dollar. They had only to permit some Japanese peasants and workers to emigrate into South American countries as they very much wanted to do.

Incidentally, why is the mortality rate in China and India, the cradle of the schools of the *tao* or the *do*, so very high? Does not such a high mortality rate among the newborn and young people in general contradict the ancient names, "country of longevity" or "medicine of the *tao*"? This is the tragic misery of peoples who have not really known the constant difficulties of hunger, heat, cold, and perpetual invasions from outside countries. The Japanese have had in the past, and have yet today, too much abundance of food. They have never really suffered from hunger. The enormous importation of food in recent years is altogether, purely and simply, a political expediency. It is ruining the people. The mortality from stomach and intestinal ailments is at its peak. That is to say, they eat too much. I and some thirty students in my institute, Centre Ignoramus (also called A New School), live on a ration of ten cents a day (one hundred percent vegetarian fare). The average person on the street spends at least seventy cents a day. The Japanese and Chinese who die young were raised according to the macrobiotic principle, but they eat great quantities of food. Quantity changes quality completely.

Principles of Freedom

Just as the people of macrobiotic countries are dying of sickness, the people of civilized countries are dying of wars. In certain countries, the average age of the people is increasing, according to statistics. But if they are not happy, if they are hemmed into a rigid society, full of fears, beset by anxiety and loneliness, what is the value of a long life? This is the condition of a prisoner with a life sentence. Crime is one barometer of the physiological health of a civilization or culture. A truly healthy person does not intentionally commit crimes. Crimes indicate serious illness. Social solidarity is in danger. This means that the leaders of the society have some grave maladies: moral myopia, spiritual color blindness, educational schizophrenia, and social and psychological sicknesses. All of these are very difficult to diagnose or even to discern, much less actually cure. The consequences of these maladies reverberate throughout society; if the leaders are spiritually sick, there will always be many sick people in society as well. Social disorder inevitably leads to complicated and grave physical sicknesses of the liver, the heart, and the kidneys.

If the statistics of a country show a high percentage of divorce, according to the words of Epictetus, this is an indication of a generally unhappy society. They do not possess the principle of harmonious unification (*musubi*) with which to establish a concrete social solidarity.

The more a police force is necessary, the more a society—as well as the individuals who are the units of that society—has no real affinity, no real connection or bond, with freedom. The more doctors and hospitals there are, the more sickness there is. Freedom is the physiognomy of a healthy society.

If someone were very strong in judo but suffered from spiritual naivete and nearsightedness, that person would be very unhappy. Such a person would eventually be scorned by society. It is the same in the case of a country. No matter how powerful a country may be, if it is lacking the principles, such as justice, that lead towards prosperity and happiness, it will soon witness the sad spectacle of its own destruction.

As Jesus said, "Seek first the kingdom of heaven and its justice." The "kingdom of heaven" is a happy society in which everybody enjoys freedom and justice one hundred percent. Justice and freedom are really the same thing, for justice is the key that makes all antagonisms become complementary.

A society with limited freedom (for example, the four freedoms as spoken of by President Roosevelt) is nonsense. The more this kind of society exists, the less there is of real freedom. I suppose you can imagine a society where the people have the four freedoms but can you imagine a society with four hundred freedoms? After all. real freedom is oneness. If that oneness of freedom is divided, it is proof that there is no understanding of it at all. This shows that its beginning, its growth and progress, its purpose, its value, its mode of existence, and its function are not understood.

Where is your freedom recorded? When and by whom? How much did it cost you? Without knowing all the conditions of freedom, one does not have the right to insist on it.

Sir Bryce, in his very important book, *Modern Democracy*, stated as such, "What is man?" When this great question has been fully elucidated, it will become possible for the first time to completely understand what democracy is. I have still not heard anyone expound on this problem clearly. Has no one yet made it clear? My dear friend the late Dr. Alexis Carrel endeavored to make this meaning clear in his famous book, *Man the Unknown*. Unfortunately, he died leaving us a new science, *The Science of Man*, incomplete.

Judo, like all other valid schools of the *do*, is for the purpose of researching oneself and resolving the enigma that has tormented human beings since ancient times: What is the human being? Aikido shows us the path we must follow. Both of these arts, in their pure form, constitute a wide door that is open to all people. Nature, society, and history are all textbooks for those who study the *do*. They become talking films that automatically unroll at any time or place.

Fabre, Seton, Lincoln, Franklin, Faraday, Erasmus, Paracelsus, Hippocrates, and Socrates were not qualified to be called real honor students in this school. They excelled rather in taking in the scenery at the side of the road and dabbling in many things. Tagore, Whitman, Thoreau, Pierre Louys, Jack London, Maupassant, Zola, Anatole France, Hugo, Handel, Wagner, Goethe, G. B. Shaw, Charles Kingsley, Samuel Butler, Shakespeare, J. J. Rousseau, Rodenbach, E. Carpenter, Georgia O'Keefe, Lewis Carroll, William Blake, Epictetus, Lao Tsu, Lenin, Stalin, Marx, and some others could rather be called the honor students of this school. Among these pupils the best were Carroll, Blake, Louys, Butler, Kingsley, Rodenbach, and O'Keefe, while Confucius, Plato, Democritus, and Locke were the lesser students. Even these lesser students, however, were still much better than the Faradays, Newton, and the so-called great men such as Kant, Hegel, Einstein, Copernicus, and da Vinci who graduated from classical schools.

What is the human being? This has been a great enigma for humanity since ancient times, a kind of invisible sphinx for those who cannot respond to this question. All animals, even a single microbe or a single animal or vegetable cell, live in total freedom. We are one kind of animal, and yet we are almost totally ignorant of the practical dialectic that is the principle of freedom. Freedom being only another word for peace, humankind is unable to live in peace. The complete freedom and happiness of all animals and vegetables living in peace can't even be compared to us. They are sometimes attacked by their natural enemies of another species, and yet they never try to injure or harm their own. They have no need for atom bombs or sophisticated weaponry. According to the opinions of Fabre, Maeterlinck, Seton, and others, they are far more moral and, above all, more honest than humans.

Peace is a state or society or world in which one lives in complete freedom without afflicting others.

Freedom is the way of living in which one does whatever one chooses, and one's actions are appreciated by everyone else also. This is accomplished without the need for any arms or instrument whatsoever and can be realized peacefully in any kind of society.

Individual peace is the spiritual quality of the person who knows that all antagonisms are also those very same complementary factors that govern over and perpetuate the universe.

World peace is a state in which a worldwide federation leads the people to, or helps them discover the way to, enjoy complete freedom without interfering or causing any disturbance in the lives of those people. This world federation governs and directs the whole society towards the establishment of a more and more elevated culture, and it does this in accordance with the principle of life—that very same principle that unifies, guides, judges, and corrects all philosophy, ideology, science, and technology. This is a universal conception, the principle of principles, the dialectical order of the universe, or more simply, the order of the universe. Concerning this principle of life, I have written over two hundred books. I sent off a score of open letters in English to one hundred and fifty world leaders. In spite of this, I have never received a single reply.

War is a reaction inevitably produced between two countries where the leaders strive to annihilate or exclude others or take up arms to preserve their wealth or monopolize their assets. Neither the leaders nor the people of such countries are aware of the dialectical conception of the universe, the key that makes antagonisms complementary.

The value of the true judo or aikido is in learning how to live a free and happy life, how to avoid dangerous situations, and how to have the dialectical principle of the order of the universe at one's beck and call. The true judo or aikido is both the actual foundation and the practice of the dialectic law of the World Federalists.

Two or three years ago, a champion American wrestler, a Mr. M., came to Japan to study judo. He could not find any judo champion able to defeat him. Finally, he went to the aikido *dojo* of Master Ueshiba; the master defeated him effortlessly. From that time on, he attended the *dojo* daily for the remaining forty days of his stay. He was staying in a first-class hotel, The Imperial. For this Western wrestler, Ueshiba's *dojo* seemed a very shabby place. One day he said to the master, "Master, come to the United States, you can become a millionaire. There is no need for you to live like this."

The master paid no attention to him whatsoever. He was in peace and freedom. Or perhaps it should be said that peace and freedom were in him. He had no desire for anything more than his present situation. In spite of his forty days of strenuous training, the wrestler nevertheless left without understanding the attitude of the master or the principle behind it. The deep ideology behind the schools of the *do* is altogether too foreign and incomprehensible for one who knows only the way of force.

Ah, now it seems that I have already said too much, and I should excuse myself. Well then, have you decided that you want to begin your study of the spirit of the *do*? Are you ready to follow in the footsteps of the true judo of Master Kano or the aikido of Master Ueshiba or his great student Mochizuki?

Quite the opposite of modern Western arts, aikido does not use much physical force. It is a technique of protecting oneself without the need for any weapon, and it employs the least possible physical force, much less still than judo. Some masters of judo are heavy; in fact, it seems that their body weight increases proportionately to the amount that they practice. The masters of aikido, however, tend to be rather lightweight and of smaller stature. It is an art that lends itself very well to women as well as men and to older people just as well as to the young. It is even possible to begin one's practice at sixty years of age or more. In this book, I have explained the principles of judo and aikido in order to show their fundamental relationship to the basis of happiness, justice, freedom, and world peace. The techniques themselves cannot be sufficiently explained with words, which are too limited in both time and space, and they also cannot be grasped by viewing photographs or watching movies of the art. They can only be understood through actual practice. It is for this reason that Mochizuki and other students of Ueshiba are already in Paris, the birthplace of many revolutionary ideas. They are all volunteers aspiring to bring about a conference of the people for a world federation.

Of course, there will always be those who will protest, saying that there is no one who can accomplish world peace or world federalism. Yet, it is not only possible, but for whoever understands the principle of life—the grandiose worldview of the infinite, dialectical construction known as the order of the universe—it is quite easy. From this view, our world, nature, and the whole of humanity is only a tiny geometric point within the infinite sea of consciousness. It is, therefore, that I repeatedly advise you, first of all, to endeavor to truly grasp the meaning of what is meant by "the order of the universe."

For those who can accomplish all their dreams completely and forever without the need for any special implement, war never did, does not now, and never will exist. These are the ones who never meet any person they do not like. They are the ones who are always loved by everyone, everywhere.

Appendix I

Afterword

If you wish to test your comprehension, memory, judgment, and adaptability using a scale of the Far East, please answer the following questions.

1. Why do humans alone use force and arms in war against their own kind? All other animals, utilizing their wonderful adaptability, fight without weapons and use only the special techniques of their own ingenuity. (See the works of Seton.)

2. How is it that humans seek to have more superior weapons and shelters than their enemies without feeling ashamed towards the animals, who use no weapons or implements whatsoever? (What appear to be weapons among some animals are only those things which God or mother nature has given them so that they may survive in their environment.)

3. Why does war exist only among human beings?

4. Why is it that people in a group will easily commit atrocities that none of them would attempt individually?

5. Why do adults unhesitatingly do things that they forbid their children to do (conduct war, for example)?

6. Why is it that some people make an image of God after the image of the physical human and yet do not attempt to equate human mentality with that of God? (If God were physically like a human being, God would be ephemeral, limited, and would certainly do very foolish things from time to time.)

7. Why is it that many leaders preach Christianity and pray in public, yet completely abandon this spirit in their private lives? Do

they pray that their enemies and the people of their own race will become Christians or do they pray for their own benefit? Why is it that they cannot "become as little children"? Do they believe that small children are stupid and of little value? Does this mean that the rest of the people and the little children should be given rat poison?

* * * * *

War is the most cruel and cowardly form of mass murder. War occurs when frightened people are led by a dictatorial government that employs ever new and increasingly effective weapons and strategy for the purpose of completely annihilating the enemy in order to protect, preserve, and increase itself. It occurs as a result of the following factors:

- Fear is the most direct and essential factor for the occurrence of war. It is a characteristic of the condition of defeatists, slaves, egoists, criminals, and those who lack as a solid foundation for their daily existence an intuitive sense of this world and the universe.
- The people, meek and obedient to dictatorial government, are mobilized for futile wars in the illusory names of justice, peace, and freedom; they are slaves ignorant of the universal constitution and are lacking a comprehensive worldview.
- The dictatorial government that drives people into war is a tool created by people who have much greater fear than other people or countries. This kind of tool is the best example of fear.
- Self-protection and self-preservation; increasing one's own sphere of influence; fear of one's own extinction; and the balance of power—all of these symbols or desires are the characteristic illusions of one who, through fear, is defeated before even beginning.

The above-mentioned fears are a kind of iron curtain that veils peace and universal understanding. Peace can only be actualized by a revolution of our concepts of biological and physiological education, the foundation of which rests within the infinite time and space of an intuitive universal conception. This universal panoramic view de-emphasizes detail. It is the antipode of modern, analytical, microscopic, electronic science, which magnifies small details.

It was the saints and the wise who succeeded in distilling this universal sense and crystallizing it into the form of yin and yang, a dialectic universal outlook or practical dialectic. The *I-Ching* was the first treatise on yin and yang. The first philosophical treatment of the subject was the *Tao Te Ching* of Lao Tsu. The *I-Ching* was later annotated and interpreted by Confucius who complicated it considerably. Nevertheless, for the past several thousand years, the principle of yin and yang has been the foundation of philosophy, the various sciences and arts, as well as the daily life of the people in China, Korea, and Japan.

I have done my best to translate it into a modern, international, and universal language. In the process of this attempt, I have completed over two hundred books and have applied this principle practically, as nutritional theory, to the food problem, the number one problem shared by all countries internationally. I have practiced it as macrobiotics and have actualized it among more than 150,000 sick and unhappy people in my clinics, sanitariums, correspondence courses, and my health institute, all of which are my *dojo* of the unifying principle.

The Order of the Universe As Logical Principles

1. Whatever has a beginning has an end (principle of invasion).

2. Whatever has a front has a back (principle of front and back).

3. There is nothing identical in this world (principle of nonduplication).

4. The bigger the front, the bigger the back (principle of balance).

5. Change (differentiation and motion) as well as stability (a momentary state of equilibrium between two fundamental, universal, dialectic, opposing, and interchanging forces) are products of yin (centrifugality) and yang (centripetality) (principle of dual origin).

6. The two conflicting forces of yin and yang are the right and left hands of the one absolute infinity (principle of polarization).

7. This great universe, the so-called world of oneness, is unchanging, limitless, constant, and omnipotent. It is infinity itself and produces, transforms, increases, destroys, and gives rebirth to all people and things both physical (*mono*) and spiritual (*koto*) (principle of polarizable monism).

Reference Notes

1. Hiroshige and Utamaro: Hiroshige Ando (1797-1858) and Utamaro Kitagawa (1753-1806) are considered among the six great masters of the Ukiyo-e school of Japanese woodblock printing. [In Japanese, the family name is first, then the given name; in this book, the reverse (English) style is used throughout. The given name only is often used for persons of honor, fame, or venerability.]

2. Lucien Lévy-Bruhl, French philosopher, sociologist, and anthropologist (1857-1939), wrote six books published between 1910 and 1938 elaborating his concept of the nature of the primitive mind and the "nonrational belief systems" of the primitive. His theories touched a responsive chord in the well-read Ohsawa, who published *Mikaijin no Seishin to Nihon Seishin* (*The Primitive Spirit and the Japanese Spirit*) in 1943 and the present volume (*Le Livre du Judo*) in 1952 in order to explain the primitive spirit from the viewpoint of a "true primitive" (himself). From his reading and personal meeting with Lévy-Bruhl, Ohsawa felt a lack of intuitive understanding on the part of the highly rational scholar.

3. Ohsawa likely took the Bible quotations in this book from a non-English source, as exact corollaries in English editions have not been found.

4. The word *macrobiotics*, anglicized from the Greek *makrobiotos* (*makro* = large + *biotis* = life), is the plural noun form of the French adjective (*macrobiotique*) adopted by Ohsawa as an equivalent to the Japanese *shokuyo* (right physical and spiritual nourishment). In the late 1700s a German physician, Christolph Wilhelm von Hufeland, used the term *makrobiotik* in reference to human longevity, although this work is not known to have been cited by Ohsawa.

5. Eugen Herrigel (1884-1955), a German professor who taught phi-

losophy at Tokyo University between the wars, penetrated deeply and personally into the theory and practice of Zen Buddhism, having trained with a Zen master for six years. Herrigel wrote two books on Zen for the Western audience, *The Method of Zen* and *Zen and the Art of Archery*, and his wife wrote a book on the art of Japanese flower arrangement (*kado*).

6. The *Manyoshu* ("Collection of a Myriad Leaves," 771 A.D.) is the oldest of the early anthologies of Japanese poetry, a reflection of Japanese life and civilization of the 7th and 8th centuries, and the greatest both in quantity and quality. It consists of 20 books containing 4,516 poems (according to the *Kokka Taikan*, Conspectus of National Poetry) written by poets of all classes who flourished in the Fujiwara and Nara periods, coinciding with the Golden Age of Chinese poetry.

7. Ohsawa refers to the 6th century Chinese treatise on strategy, a compilation translated as the Seven Canons (or Articles) of War. See note #20.

8. The Meiji Restoration (*Meiji Ishin*, the Meiji era renovation), also known as the Great Meiji Reform: The great social, political, and economic reforms of Japan following a palace coup on January 3,1868, in which a group of nobles and samurai seized the Imperial Palace in Kyoto and demanded the formal return of political power from the Tokugawa Shogunate to the emperor. Following a brief civil war (the Boshin War), national unity was achieved by spring 1869 under Emperor Meiji.

9. World Federalism began in the United States after the war (1947), proposing a world government on a federal basis with powers of maintaining order and peace among the nations. Ohsawa joined the movement, becoming a leader of the Japanese branch in 1948; his study center (Maison Ignoramus) in Yokohama was given a second name, "The World Government Center," and he began publishing a biweekly newspaper called *Sekai Seifu* (World Government). Ohsawa succeeded to some extent in combining his macrobiotic views with the principles of the movement. Norman Cousins, World Federalist leader in America and founder of *The Saturday Review of Literature*, visited the Yokoha-

ma center for a week. Interestingly, Cousins's writing during the 1980s turned towards personal health issues.

10. Gresham's Law: The observation in economics that "bad money drives out good." If two coins have the same nominal value but are made from metals of unequal value, the cheaper will tend to drive the other out of circulation. Sir Thomas Gresham (1518-1579), financial agent of Queen Elizabeth I, was not the first to observe this principle, but his elucidation of it in 1558 prompted the economist H. D. Macleod to suggest the term "Gresham's Law" in the 19th century. (From the *Encyclopedia Brittanica.*)

11. Romain Rolland (1866-1944), novelist, dramatist, essayist, and one of the great mystics of 20th century French literature, was deeply involved in the major social, political, and spiritual events of his time, including pacifism and the search for world peace. An interpreter of Eastern philosophy to the West, as was Ohsawa, Rolland is the subject of Chapter 7 in Ohsawa's *Jack and Mitie in the West* (George Ohsawa Macrobiotic Foundation, 1981). The two met in Paris around 1930.

12. Son of a samurai trader in Yokohama, art critic and philosopher Kakuzo Okakura (1862-1913), more commonly known by his pen name Tenshin, wrote the celebrated *The Book of Tea*, published in 1906. Eventually becoming assistant curator of the Chinese and Japanese Department of the Boston Museum of Fine Arts, his exhibits, lectures, and publications were designed to educate the West about Asian culture. Okakura's books were widely read in English and his ideas strongly influenced Western perceptions of Japanese culture.

13. Edmond (1822-1896) and Jules (1830-1870) Goncourt, wealthy Parisian brothers, were art collectors, novelists, and historians who wrote documentary novels and monographs on art and history. Edmond did much to awaken interest in Japanese art in Europe, particularly the artists Utamaro and Hokusai.

14. Charles Peguy (1873-1914), French essayist and poet. A Socialist, nationalist, and mystical Catholic remaining outside the Church,

his writing style features constant repetition, bearing a parallel to Oh-sawa's.

15. Pierre Louys (1870-1925), born in Ghent of French parents, was a novelist and poet, member of the Symbolists, writer on life in ancient Greece, and founder of two exclusive literary reviews.

16. Lafcadio Hearn (1850-1904) was one of the most prolific writers in English in transmitting aspects of Japanese culture to the Western audience. *Japan, an Attempt at Interpretation*, post-humously published, is his most famous work. Born in the Ionian Islands to Greek and British parents, he taught English literature at Tokyo University until 1903. Having married into a Japanese family, he became a naturalized Japanese citizen and took the name Yakumo Koizumi. Hearn had also met Jigoro Kano, founder of Kodokan Judo, and in 1897 published a chapter entitled "Jiujitsu" in his *Out of the East—Reveries and Studies in New Japan* (Charles E. Tuttle Company, 1977).

17. Cited by Ohsawa as a Western thinker who understood the Eastern mind, F. S. C. Northrop (1893-1992) was born in England and was named Sterling Professor of Philosophy and Law Emeritus, Yale University, in 1962. *The Meeting of East and West* was published in 1946 and subsequently translated into Japanese by Ohsawa, who felt it was one of the most significant writings of the 20th century.

18. This refers to the assassination of the shogunal great elder Nao-suke Ii-tairo outside Sakurada Gate of Edo (Tokyo) Castle on March 24, 1860 by anti-shogunate activists. This led to the eventual overthrow of the shogunate (1867-68) and the beginning of the Meiji Restoration. *Tairo* means "great elder," the highest ranking position below the shogun in the Tokugawa Shogunate (1603-1867). Until 1867, only lords of the Ii family held the title. "Taira" is a family name, one of the four great families related to the imperial family dominating court politics during the Heian period (794-1185).

19. Basis of Kano's Kodokan Judo: *Seiryoku Zenyo*, "The Principle of the Best Use of Physical and Spiritual Energy," as well as *Jita Kyoei*,

"The Principle of Mutual Welfare." (*Asian Fighting Arts*, by Donn F. Draeger, instructor at Kodokan, Tokyo, and Robert W. Smith. Medallion Books, New York, 1974.)

20. The Taoist idea that one should be inwardly firm and strong (yang) while outwardly soft and flexible (yin), fundamental in Ohsawa's teaching, is stressed in Sun Tsu's classic of military strategy, *The Art of War* (*Sun-tsu ping fa*, China, 500 B.C.; in Japanese, *Heiho Shichisho, The Seven Articles of War*). Permeated with the philosophy of Lao Tsu and the *Tao Te Ching*, the treatise contains the principle that "The supreme art of war is to subdue the enemy without fighting," the ultimate goal of judo and aikido.

21. Paul Ehrlich (1854-1915), German biologist, shared the Nobel prize in 1908 for his work with Metchnikoff on immunology. Walther Flemming (18434905), German cell scientist and researcher, coined the term *mitosis* for indirect cell division. Frederick Grant Banting (1891-1941), Canadian endocrinologist, won the 1923 Nobel prize in physiology/medicine for his early animal (pancreatic) experiments that led to the commercial production of insulin for treating diabetes (in 1922). C. H. Best was his collaborator.

22. Maison Ignoramus ("Ignoramus house") was the name Ohsawa gave to his live-in study center established just after the war, in 1947. The school was like a *dojo*, practice center for a spiritual discipline; it was here that future macrobiotic leaders such as Cornellia Aihara, Aveline Kushi, Herman Aihara, and Michio Kushi received their training from Ohsawa. To this day, the Paris macrobiotic center publishes a periodical called *Ignoramus*, and in Tokyo the International Macrobiotic Center is known as the C.I., or Centre Ignoramus. During his world travels and in Japan, Ohsawa brought his "spiritual *dojo*" with him under the name of A New School, or A.N.S. This sometimes took the form of months-long outdoor camps, setting a model for the worldwide macrobiotic summer camps of today.

23. In his near-Stoic recommendation for living the simple life, Ohsawa often used this Latin phrase in his writing. Albius Tibullus, a Roman

elegiac poet who died about B.C. 18, used the phrase "Possim contentus vivere parvo" in one of his poems (Tibullus 1, 1, 25), literally, "May I be capable of being content with just a little." In Horace's *Odes* (2, 16, and 13) one finds "Vivitur parvo bene," or "One can live well with little." In the first line of Horace's Satires, Book II, Number 2, one finds: "Quae virtus et quanta, boni, sit vivere parvo." Jim Poggi, editor of the English version of Ohsawa's *The Order of the Universe* (George Ohsawa Macrobiotic Foundation, 1986), suggests the following interpretation: "How completely empowering it can be, my good friends, to make do with as little as possible."

24. The reference here is to Caspar Milquetoast, the American cartoon character created by H. T. Webster in 1924. "Milquetoast" came to signify a timid or unforthcoming person, based on the character's portrayal. According to Herman Aihara, Ohsawa was fond of the term.

25. Ernest Thompson Seton (1860-1946), English-born American writer and illustrator. Jean-Henri Fabre (1823-1915), French entomologist. Maurice, Polydore, and Marie-Bernard Maeterlinck (circa 1862-1949), Belgian poets/dramatists/essayists.

26. Robert Falcon Scott (1868-1912), English explorer. Fridtjof Nansen (1861-1930), Norwegian arctic explorer, zoologist, and statesman.

27. Sir James Bryce (1838-1922), British jurist, historian, and diplomat, author of *Modern Democracy*.

28. Alexis Carrel (1873-1944), French surgeon and biologist, and author. Ohsawa often cited Carrel's work and translated his *Man, The Unknown* (*L'Homme Inconnu*) from French to Japanese through a major Japanese publishing house. Ohsawa found in the distinguished scientist and winner of the 1923 Nobel prize for medicine a kindred spirit in criticizing Western science and technology.

29. Musashi Miyamoto (1584-1645), illustrious samurai swordmaster of the Tokugawa era, wrote the classic *Go Rin No Sho* (*A Book of Five Rings*) just before his death as a final treatise on strategy. The English translation by Victor Harris (Overtook Press, New York, 1974) became

an American bestseller and, like Sun Tsu's *The Art of War*, is interpreted allegorically for business or philosophy as well as martial strategy. Ohsawa's quotation appears to have been paraphrased from the second chapter, "The Water Book."

30. The book, published in English entitled *Nagasaki 1945* (Quartet Books Limited, London, 1981), was written by Dr. Tatsuichiro Akizuki, president of St. Francis Hospital, Nagasaki, Japan.

31. Ellsworth Huntington (1876-1947), American geographer and explorer, author of *Climate and Civilization* (Yale University Press, New Haven, revised 1924).

32. Edward Carpenter (1844-1929), English writer and Anglican clergyman who left the Church after becoming interested in the Socialist and crafts movements. Carpenter met Emerson and Whitman in the United States in 1877 and published *Civilization, Its Cause and Cure* in 1889, suggesting activity and diet for health maintenance.

Glossary
of Japanese Terms

AIKIDO: Martial arts form developed in Japan (1942) by Morihei Ueshiba with techniques based on natural rhythm and nonresistance. AIKIDO (*ai* – coordinate; *ki* – spirit; *do* – way) or *aiki-jujutsu* (Ohsawa refers to "aiki-judo") emerged as a second eclectic system from JU-JUTSU. The other is JUDO.

AZUKI: Small red bean, highly regarded in Japan for its nutritional and strengthening qualities, often used as a folk remedy.

BUDO: From *bushido* (*bu* – military; *shi* – knight; *do* – way), the unwritten code of morals or chivalry among the warrior (samurai) class of old Japan.

CHADO: The art of the Japanese tea ceremony (*cha* – tea; *do* – way). Also *sado*.

DAIMYO: Feudal lord or baron, advisor to the shogun (rulers of Japan prior to 1867).

DAN: Step, level, or grade among practitioners of martial arts.

DO: Way, art, or practice.

DOJO: Practice or exercise hall or gymnasium. Place where the way (*do*) is studied.

GEIDO: The way of art or artistic accomplishments.

GETA: High wooden clogs worn outdoors, known in Japan as early as 300 B.C.

GOKUI: The highest teaching of principle and technique.

HAKAMA: Formal ceremonial skirts worn by boys and men of the samurai class.

IDO: The way of medicine.

JUDO: Martial arts form synthesized in Japan (1882) by Jigoro Kano emphasizing the correct way and time to resist or yield to an opponent. JUDO (*ju* – soft or supple; *do* – way) is the first eclectic system that took the place of the earlier JUJUTSU. The second is AIKIDO.

JUJITSU: Also JUJUTSU (or *jiujitsu* or *jiujutsu*): Generic term applied to 725 officially documented systems of armed or unarmed combat based on flexibility and yielding instead of force (*ju* – soft or yielding; *jutsu* – art or means).

KADO: The Japanese art of flower arrangement, now generally known as *ikebana*, originating in the 6th century with the introduction of Buddhism from China.

KANGAERU: Japanese verb "to think." Ohsawa wrote that KANGAERU thinking (as opposed to OMOU) refers to things that are infinite and absolute (freedom, happiness, justice, etc.).

KATSU: To win, as in a battle.

KENDO: The way of the sword; Japanese fencing based on the techniques of the two-handed sword of the samurai, implying spiritual discipline as well as fencing technique. Before the Showa period (1926-1989), it was referred to as *kenjutsu* (*ken* – sword; *jutsu* – art) or gekken.

KODOKAN: The name of the DOJO established in 1882 by Jigoro Kano for the practice of JUDO. KODOKAN JUDO refers to the form, the DOJO, and the educational foundation for the teaching and promotion of JUDO in Tokyo.

KOKUSHI: Administrators of Japanese provinces (provincial governors) in the Nara period (710-794).

KOTO: Ideas; inspirational things or meanings.

KUDEN: Oral teaching or instruction.

KYUDO: Japanese archery, the way of the bow. *Kyujutsu* was the term in use until the late 19th century.

MAKOTO: Truth or reality in the absolute sense.

MICHI: Way or path. Synonymous with *do*, but the common usage is more physical, as in road or street.

MIKAN: Tangerine-like citrus fruit grown profusely in Japan, known as Satsuma or mandarin orange.

MONO: Physical things or objects.

MONO NO FU: Samurai warrior.

MUSUBI: United, joined; meanings also include knot or tie (as in the marriage bond) and rice-ball.

OKUGI: The highest teaching of a school (*do*).

OMOTE-URA: Front and back; surface and reverse.

OMOU: Japanese verb "to think" or "consider." Ohsawa wrote that OMOU thinking (as opposed to KANGAERU) refers to things that are finite and relative (money, power, knowledge, etc.).

SENPAI (or *Sempai*): Senior student or graduate of the same school.

SENSEI: Teacher or instructor, often applied to professor, doctor, or person of knowledge.

SHIHAN: Master (also teacher or instructor), often applied to master of an art, such as a fencing master.

SHIN: True or real in the factual sense.

SHINGON: Major sect of Buddhism, the esoteric sect founded by Kukai in the early 9th century.

SHINTO: The indigenous Japanese national religion. A complex system of religious practices and ideas crystallized during the Nara (710-794) and Heian (794-1185) periods; in dynamic interaction with other Asian religious systems (Buddhism, Taoism, and Confucianism).

SHODO: Calligraphy, the way (*do*) of brush-writing (*sho*).

SHOJIN RYORI: Vegetarian cooking or diet derived from imperial court cuisine, developed by monks and nuns in Buddhist temples of the early Zen sects.

SHUGYU: Spiritual training or practice in search of enlightenment.

SUNAO: As adjectival form *sunao na*: Obedient, meek, or gentle.

TAO: Chinese rendering of DO (way). In Taoist philosophy, the creative principle that orders the universe.

TATAMI: Rush-covered straw flooring mats about 2.4 inches thick, used in traditional Japanese-style rooms. Also a standard unit of measure, approximately 3 by 6 feet.

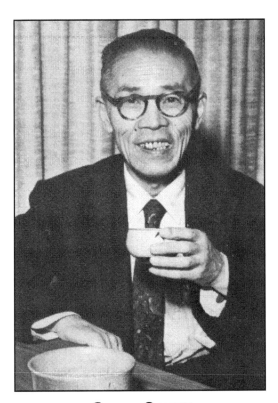

GEORGE OHSAWA

About the Author

George Ohsawa (Nyoichi Sakurazawa, 1893-1966) was born in Kyoto, the old capital of Japan, at a time when Japan had only recently opened its doors culturally and economically to the rest of the world. Enduring family hardships and frail health as a youth, Ohsawa encountered the *shokuyo* system of health formulated in the late 1800s by Sagen Ishizuka, a scholar and physician integrating many ancient sources of traditional wisdom. With Ishizuka's method, he was able to heal his pulmonary tuberculosis before the age of twenty.

From this point on, Ohsawa remained devoted to the advancement of this system, renamed *macrobiotics*, and with his wife Lima he travelled worldwide with his message, staying for extended periods in India, Africa, France, Vietnam, and the United States.

As Ohsawa brought physical techniques and understanding to the Western world, he also brought aspects of Asian culture, thought, and spirituality. In France and the United States, he imparted many of the Japanese arts and practices, including judo and aikido, that have enriched society and provided a bridge between East and West. No less passionately, he introduced elements of Western culture to the East, translating important works from French and English to Japanese.

For his wartime efforts as a peace activist, Ohsawa narrowly escaped execution by firing squad and was imprisoned for the greater part of 1945.

A list of books by George Ohsawa and others on macrobiotics can be obtained from the George Ohsawa Macrobiotic Foundation, PO Box 3998, Chico, CA 95927-3998; 530-566-9765; fax 530-566-9768; *gomf@earthlink.net*. Or, visit *www.ohsawamacrobiotics.com*.